A SHEARWATER BOOK

Lake Effect

Lake Effect

Two Sisters and
a Town's Toxic Legacy

NANCY A. NICHOLS

ISLANDPRESS / Shearwater Books
Washington • Covelo • London

Library of Congress Cataloging-in-Publication data.

Nichols, Nancy A., 1959–
Lake effect : two sisters and a town's toxic
legacy / by Nancy A. Nichols.
p. cm.
Includes bibliographical references and index.
ISBN-13: 978-1-59726-084-8 (cloth : alk. paper)
ISBN-10: 1-59726-084-3 (cloth : alk. paper)
1. Cancer—Environmental aspects—Illinois—Waukegan.
2. Polychlorinated biphenyls—Environmental aspects—
Illinois—Waukegan. I. Title.
RC268.25.N53 2009
616.99'40710977321—DC22   2008010305

British Cataloguing-in-Publication data available.

Printed on recycled, acid-free paper ♻
Design by Joyce C. Weston
Manufactured in the United States of America

10 9 8 7 6 5 4 3 2 1

Keywords: health, industrial pollution, Superfund sites,
memoir, Great Lakes, pancreatic cancer, ovarian cancer,
PCBs, endometriosis, endocrine disruptors

Contents

Lake Michigan is known for its deep, cold waters and for the powerful storms it brews. Known as the "lake effect," snow that piles up as far away as Buffalo can be traced to the bitter cold air that drives across the lake gathering speed and humidity.

I grew up on the shores of the lake in the heavily industrialized town of Waukegan, Illinois. In spring and summer, thunderstorms blew off the one-hundred-mile-wide lake, driving wind and rain toward our town and sending debris swirling across yards and roads. Frequent tornado warnings would send us into the basement, our knees knocking under our skirts with anxiety. In winter, storms brought icy winds and heavy snowfalls that pummeled us as we walked to and from school.

Given the power of the lake to shape weather miles away, I suppose it should not have come as a surprise that the volatile, beautiful body of water at the edge of my town would play a role in my family too. It did, but many years would pass before we felt its full effect.

CHAPTER ONE

The Used-Car Salesman's Daughters

IN THE AFTERMATH OF my mother's death when I was ten years old, my older sister became a kind of substitute Mom. To console me that first summer, we often went as a big sister/little sister dyad to the Lake Michigan shore.

The municipal beach in Waukegan was a small piece of land edged by factories and the town's water processing plant. If you were facing the lake when the sun rose, our town beach looked like a picture postcard; but at sunset the string of factories cast long shadows over the bandstand, the snack shop, and the playground.[1] The factories did not deter us, however. Like so many townspeople, we simply turned our back on them and enjoyed the lake.

My sister had a small yellow bikini and ultrawhite skin. I was tanned brown and sticky from candy or ice cream or both. She was nineteen, drove a red Mustang, and had a beehive hairdo. She had perfect penmanship, scratched out with a thin blue fountain pen. Everything about me was messy or dirty or untamed in comparison.

Part sister, part mother, part friend, Sue handed me my first tampon, taught me how to shave my legs, and told me about sex—although I later used to tease her that I never quite had the earth-shaking, sheet-rattling experience that she summoned up in our less than scientific little chats. "How do you do that again?" I would ask, and she would blush and shove me away, saying, "Shut up."

We were the daughters of a used-car salesman who was notable mostly for having once sold more Dodge Darts than any other man in the state. At nearly six foot four, my father dressed the part of a car salesman as well as he played it. He was unmistakable in his lime green leisure suits with white belts. His slicked-back white hair was a perfect match for his black shirts with white ties and checkerboard sports jackets.

Our father lied about everything, consistently, reflexively. It was an occupational hazard. He lied about unimportant, useless things, like which grocery store he went to; and about enormous things too, like whether or not the car was insured or whether there was oil in the furnace. He lied about which branch of the service he had been in during World War II, as if that would matter to anyone. He lied about having gone to college, which he never did. I don't know whether he had always lied and that made him an excellent car salesman or whether he started lying once he started selling cars and then adopted it as a lifestyle.

No matter. Our father's unceasing lying caused us to crave the definitive. We were fact-crazed girls who grew into hard-bitten realists as women. My sister became a title searcher—someone who checks that the property you are about to buy is owned wholly by the seller with no outstanding liens. She made sure that all was in order, recording transaction after transaction on three-by-five-inch cards in the days before personal computers, carefully sorting and storing them in the closet. I worked as a reporter, hunting for little facts that taken together might prove some larger truth.

After we reached adulthood, she moved farther out into the county, just west of Waukegan, and I went off first to college and then to New York and Boston to pursue a career in magazines and television. Though from different vantage points, we both avidly followed the news from our hometown.

When I was in high school in the late 1970s, sporadic reports of contaminants near the beach and in the harbor had already begun to appear. After we left town, the slow trickle of stories became a torrent, eventually landing Waukegan on the front page of national newspapers and on the network news. As the story evolved, my sister and I traded newspaper clippings and studied reports that named the sources of the pollutants and identified the chemicals that had suffused our early years without our knowledge.

In long, late-night phone calls, news of the contaminants mixed with news of what my sister was wearing, what kind of curtains she should get for her bedroom, and what she was making for dinner. On trips back home in the late 1980s, we walked the borders of the restricted zones together, peering around fences emblazoned with skull and crossbones near childhood haunts. The farm where we bought our vegetables, restaurants we frequented, and the nursing home where my grandmother lived all ringed one site that was less than a mile from our home. As we toured the places of our childhood, the scope of the pollution seeped into our consciousness in the same way that it had slowly slipped into the groundwater.

I don't think it occurred to either of us in those years that we might personally be affected by what had been discovered in the sediment, the groundwater, even in the lake itself. It didn't occur to us, that is, until 1992, when my sister was diagnosed with a rare form of ovarian cancer. She was only forty-one at the time, and there was only a minimal history of cancer in our family. We both began to wonder aloud whether there could be a link between the chemical contamination in our hometown and her cancer. And once the seed of that possibility was planted, our curiosity took root.

It was late the next year that my sister, weak and failing from chemotherapy and a bone-marrow transplant, whispered to me in the same secretive tone she had used to explain everything—sex, the death of our mother, and most recently in the tiniest voice imaginable, her cancer—"You have to write about this." I knew what she wanted. She wanted me to make meaning out of her agony, to make sure that all her suffering would amount to something in the end.

"I will," I assured her as I ran my hand over the thin hair on her head. I called her little ducky head because of the soft, downy hair that she grew between rounds of chemotherapy. "You're beautiful."

"Am not, and you shouldn't say it."

"Are too," I said as I stroked her arm. She gave a little half smile and went back to sleep.

If she had been feeling better, I would have argued, "No, don't be stupid. Get up. Write your own book." Instead, I murmured, "Don't worry, I can do it," as I tucked the covers under her chin. I made the promise the same way I might have told her she could borrow my sweater. I knew what she wanted, but I never expected I would have to deliver. I had hoped then—had even believed at some level—that she would get up and get better.

My sister was my biggest fan, and even in her chemo-induced haze she argued that I could write the kind of book she imagined. As a journalist working in print and television, I had covered some of the major environmental stories of the 1980s, stories that led to conversations that, in turn, would cause us to wonder about our hometown. In 1982, in Times Beach, Missouri, for example, investigators had discovered that oil tinged with a dangerous chemical called dioxin had been sprayed on the floors of horse stables and on dirt roads to manage dust. A river flood then washed dioxin-contaminated soil into homes. Eventually, the federal government bought out homeowners and businesses in a large-scale resettlement.[2]

Waukegan would take its turn on the national stage two years later, in 1984, when a U.S. Environmental Protection Agency official, Rita Lavelle, was accused of secretly meeting with lakefront polluters in an effort to strike a cleanup deal that heavily favored industry. Lavelle was forced to resign when a congressional committee discovered her inappropriate backdoor negotiations and other transgressions.

In the aftermath of the scandal, the full extent of Waukegan's chemical contamination was revealed. By far the largest single source of pollution on the lakefront, and the first identified, was the one million pounds of sediment contaminated with polychlorinated biphenyls (PCBs) lining the town's harbor. These fire- and pressure-resistant substances were banned as possible cancer-causing chemicals in 1976, a year before I graduated from high school and the same year that lakefront pollution was first investigated by state and federal authorities.[3]

Eventually, three separate Superfund sites, named after the 1980 federal legislation that allocated funds to clean them up, were designated in Waukegan. Two of the sites are adjacent to the lake. The other is a landfill—less than a mile from our childhood home—where many of the industrial pollutants from the manufacturing facilities on the lake were trucked. In addition, more than a dozen other sites form what federal and state regulators call an expanded study area, which stretches along the lakefront from one end of town to the other. These smaller sites contain the waste products from a tannery, a steel company, a paint factory, a pharmaceutical company, and a scrap yard. Together, these sites contain not just PCBs, but an alphabet soup of pollutants.

"Just about every chemical we know to be dangerous to human health is in one of those sites," says Margaret Quinn, a professor at the University of Massachusetts, Lowell, who specializes in human exposure assessment.[4] In addition to PCBs, these chemicals include benzene and other volatile organic compounds, arsenic, lead, asbestos, polycyclic aromatic hydrocarbons (PAHs), dioxins, vinyl chloride, and ammonia. Various chemicals among these have been associated with reproductive diseases, learning and attention deficits in children, birth defects, immune system deficiencies, and some forms of cancer.

Was there a relationship between my sister's cancer and the toxins of our childhood? My sister certainly thought so. And many other people have suspected, often correctly, that elements in their environment have had an effect on their health. Yet because of the long time it takes for a cancer to develop and because of the relative mobility of our lives today, it can be challenging to establish a causal link between a disease and its origin.

In my hometown, for example, the factories that lined the lake when I was a child are for the most part boarded up and bankrupt, some have been torn down and carted away, and only a few remain active. Much of Waukegan's present population is new to the area; the men who worked in those plants and their children have passed away or have scattered in search of better jobs and cleaner towns.

In order to fulfill my promise to my sister, then, I could not simply comb the town looking for other people who might be sick, piecing together patterns observed along the way. I would need to stitch my story together from a variety of sources. I made repeated visits to my hometown to find out what I could there, of course. But I also hired researchers to help me understand the technical literature, I read and reread studies of the effects of toxins, and I interviewed experts. I studied the chemicals in the lake and the processes that scientists believe lead to cancer. And I talked to the men I could locate who had managed the factories.

I spoke, for example, to the person who used to run the Johns-Manville plant that produced asbestos-laden building products on Waukegan's lakefront. Asbestos is a natural substance that when inhaled can cause a severe and deadly lung cancer called malignant mesothelioma. Every single member of his administrative staff had died, he told me. Workers' health claims from the Waukegan plant and elsewhere grew to hundreds of millions of dollars. In a controversial move, Johns-Manville filed for bankruptcy in 1982, seeking to protect the company from the growing stack of liability claims. The company was later reorganized, but the Waukegan plant closed permanently.

This story was repeated again and again in Waukegan and in similar communities around the Great Lakes and elsewhere. The industries along the lake fell like dominoes in the wake of environmental and health concerns, or they moved away or were simply driven under by poor management and increasing foreign competition. Waukegan lost close to thirty-five thousand jobs in the three decades between the 1970s, when extensive pollution was officially documented, and 2001, when the final polluter on the lakefront went bankrupt.

With the resulting working-class diaspora and other population changes went any chance of a large-scale epidemiological study to document the effects of toxic exposure in Waukegan's residents and plant workers. Indeed, statistics for the town and surrounding area don't show any incidence of cancer or other diseases beyond what might be expected in the general population. But I know these statistics are misleading because they don't include the men who have already died from exposure to asbestos and the people who simply moved away when the jobs left.

Cancer is, of course, a complicated illness. In some instances, genetic heredity is an overwhelming factor. But there are many external factors that can lead to or influence the disease, such as toxins both man-made and natural in our food, water, and air. And then there is the body's sophisticated and distinct response to invasive toxins. The strength of a person's immune system, an individual's genetic makeup, and perhaps even a person's stress level can affect how, or if, disease develops. It is a complex dance between an individual and his or her environment that leads to disease. What evidence was there about the toxins in my town? What role might they play in serious human illnesses such as my sister's?

Although I set out to write an account of one person's illness, what I found was a universal story. Some of the toxic chemicals in my hometown are banned now, but they are still present in many places—and they are similar in both their structural composition and effect to many other chemicals that remain in use today, accumulating in our bodies and those of our loved ones. All of us have a lifetime of toxic exposures to contend with—from air, from water, from the food we eat. The amount of exposure, its timing, and the particular mix of the chemical cocktail we have each ingested are all relevant to our own health and the health of our children.

Studies show that many people today, even those living in remote areas of the world, carry an enormous body burden of chemical substances. Persistent chemicals similar to the type that we encountered in Waukegan can be found in the bloodstreams of those who live in urban industrialized areas and those who live in rural and remote lands. These toxins are present in the bodies of the Inuit people living on the rim of the Arctic and in the bodies of the wealthiest women living privileged lives in California. Elderly people carry caches of toxins in their bodies, and the youngest among us who ingest a mother's stored contaminants in breast milk can show the highest concentration of pollutants.

Studies by both the U.S. Environmental Protection Agency and the Centers for Disease Control and Prevention have found measurable levels of industrial chemicals in *all* adults tested in the United States. No longer is it necessary to spend your summer days lolling on the beach near a toxic-waste site as my sister and I did to end up with a hefty dose of industrial chemicals. In 2007, the American Cancer Society, for example, listed more than two hundred chemicals found commonly in urban air and everyday consumer products that are capable of producing breast cancer in animals.[5] Where once we thought of pollution simply as existing outside of us—in the landfill, or in the lake, or in the lagoon behind the factory—today it's recognized that each and every one of us is a walking environment, and often a toxic one at that.

The feedback loops created by what we produce, how we produce it, and how and where we store the wastes created in the process can be found over and over again in our society. As we change the land and the landscape, it changes us. "As humans have industrialized the land, the land has, in turn, industrialized them," writes the environmental historian Linda Nash in *Inescapable Ecologies*. "Neither the realm of nature nor the realm of the human remains pure."[6] Nowhere did this perverse relationship between ourselves, the industries we create, the environment we often neglect, and our health play out more clearly than in my hometown and in my family.

CHAPTER TWO

Green Town

ᐒ

RAY BRADBURY, THE NOTED science fiction writer and novelist, was born in Waukegan in 1920 and spent part of his childhood there. In his 1957 novel *Dandelion Wine*, he painted an idealized picture of the place, even naming it Green Town. By the time I was growing up there, however, the town was anything but green.

For Bradbury, Waukegan was a vibrant town with rain barrels and grape arbors and spent firecrackers lying on dew-kissed lawns. Verdant trees touched as they arched over the top of streets, bees with feet dusted by hundreds of blossoms buzzed happily, and boys rollicked in deep ravines. Bradbury's romanticized version of the town, however, belied its long commercial history. Nestled along Lake Michigan's shores almost precisely halfway between Chicago and Milwaukee, Waukegan has been a site for commerce since a well-known Jesuit missionary, Jacques Marquette, arrived in 1673 and established a trading fort. Just over two hundred years later, in 1885, the bustling little town with a population of just over four thousand boasted several breweries, tanneries, and mills and a mattress factory.[1]

By the time Bradbury was born there thirty-five years later, the town had added a coking plant, a paint factory, and a steel company to the long list of factories along the lake. Instead of focusing on Waukegan's growing industrial presence, though, Bradbury chose to write about the town's rich natural setting, a setting that would become little more than a tragic backdrop to the incessant industrialization and toxic outpourings that characterized my childhood in the town.

The physical features that captured Bradbury's attention—the lake, the bluffs, and the deep ravines that run through town—were carved out by glaciers at the end of the ice age. The Waukegan River, barely more than a trickle in some places, runs through town and empties into the lake. The area just south of where the harbor is today was once among the most productive fishing spots in all the Great Lakes, known for its record hauls of perch and whitefish.

Waukegan was not a natural port, however. There was no inlet or naturally protected area to serve as a harbor. As a result, locals eager to grab a portion of the trade that passed offshore between Chicago and Milwaukee improvised. At first they simply built three piers out into the lake. Then, in 1852, Congress approved $15,000 for a breakwater, though that structure washed away in one of Lake Michigan's legendary storms.[2] In 1881, Congress appropriated another $15,000 and work began anew. "It was not a simple job," writes William Ashworth in *The Late, Great Lakes*. "There were no natural openings in the coastline in the Waukegan vicinity."[3] Still, the determined people of the town dug a harbor into the sand at a cost of about $225,000 in the early 1900s.

The new harbor and the accommodating adjacent flats lured business on an ever larger scale. Commonwealth Edison built a coal-fired generating station in Waukegan in 1920 that still operates today. Johns-Manville completed its plant for manufacturing asbestos-laced roofing and other building materials in 1922.4 Five years later, in 1927, the company whose legacy would include one million pounds of PCB-contaminated sediment in the Waukegan harbor—the Johnson Motors Company, a division of the Outboard Marine Corporation—completed its $1.25 million plant.5

Waukegan's natural amenities and new harbor had clearly attracted new industries—what better place to test boat motors, after all, than on the lake?—but there was an additional lure. Waukegan's new plants were far from the unionized activities and labor unrest that plagued Chicago at the time.6 Nonunion workers, who were by and large recent European émigrés from Lithuania, Slovenia, and Armenia, staffed these newly completed factories and eventually settled into Waukegan. Articles from the *Waukegan Daily Sun* in the 1920s also report that the factories "imported negroes" as workers from the South.7

With the needs of industry satiated, at least temporarily, legislation to save a portion of the land just north of the factories began in the 1920s. In 1948, the area was turned into a four-thousand-acre preserve named Illinois Beach State Park.8 But Waukegan's fate had been sealed by the large-scale factories whose very production processes ensured that they would also become large-scale polluters. As Rachel Carson put it in *Silent Spring*, "The history of life on earth has been a history of the interaction between living things and their surroundings."9 Waukegan would be no different.

The harbor's development created a "sweet spot" for the town. It attracted both fishermen and industry in a mix that would at first spur economic growth, but would later prove disastrous. Fishermen enjoyed great catches three seasons a year and manufacturing jobs during the winter when they were unable to fish. Manufacturers enjoyed a unique location accessible to an important rail line and the harbor. As these advantages became known, the town grew steadily, with both industry and commercial fishing booming.

The town's population increased all through the 1950s and 1960s, largely because of newcomers arriving to work in the booming factories.[10] By the late 1960s, the town's population was more than sixty-five thousand and the town's 130 factories produced more than 450 different products.[11] A 1967 newspaper editorial emphasized the rapid increase in the number of jobs, noting that the median annual household income in Waukegan had been $9,437 the previous year (roughly $60,000 a year in today's dollars). This was a living wage that supported good public schools and a robust community life.

For the mayor of Waukegan in those decades, Robert Sabonjian, jobs were both part of his vision for the town and a tool he used to wield political power. As one political scientist put it, "Sabonjian believes that the prosperity and stability of his city depend upon a high rate of employment."[12] Job growth also allowed Sabonjian to consolidate his political power by rewarding the loyal. "If somebody wants a job," Sabonjian would say, "I'll find him one." So many job seekers showed up at one plant's personnel office with a letter from the mayor that those who came empty-handed were sent to the mayor's office to get one.

Sabonjian's power was legendary. A Democrat, he was often likened to Mayor Richard Daley of Chicago—except that many people thought Sabonjian had more power.[13] There were persistent rumors that Sabonjian was corrupt, and his own bragging sometimes fueled the rumor mill. "He freely talks about the gifts—boats, cars and free lunches—that businesses and industries have given him in return for things the city has done for them," wrote Kenan Heise and Edward Baumann in *Chicago Originals*.[14] Yet a five-month-long federal grand jury investigation into charges of corruption and misconduct failed to return any indictments.

One thing was clear: Sabonjian was a friend to business and saw economic growth as paramount. This growth would be good for the town in many ways through the 1960s and 1970s and even into the early 1980s. Taxes on steady factory wages built good schools and a strong community. The strategy would backfire, however, when vast amounts of pollutants were officially "discovered" in the 1970s after locals began to complain of drinking water with an unusual medicinal taste and anglers reported strange deformities in fish caught in the lake.

In the 1980s and 1990s, factories along the lake closed one by one—victims of increased regulation, high costs of court-ordered cleanups, foreign competition, poor management, and outdated technologies. When the factories closed, the workers left, or, in the case of asbestos workers, they died with hard, hacking coughs. Workers from Waukegan had over one hundred asbestos-related health claims pending when the Johns-Manville Corporation filed for bankruptcy in August 1982 in a bid to shield itself from further liability claims.[15]

Just down the road, the Outboard Marine Corporation—the company that was the source of the PCBs in the lake—closed its plant in the late 1990s. When local reporters asked the company spokeswoman, Marlena Cannon, in 1998 whether there was any hostility over all the damage that had been done to the lake and town, she gave her own spin, saying, "That was years ago, all that is forgotten."[16]

I suppose it is over for some people, but for Ray Bradbury and for me, this story is far from finished. Bradbury published a sequel to *Dandelion Wine* in 2006, titled *Farewell Summer*. Nearly eighty years after he was born there, Bradbury is still captivated by his hometown. So am I.

Waukegan certainly has not lived up to Bradbury's idyllic vision, and I am not the first to notice. One writer quipped that Waukegan could not win a beauty contest even if the only other contestant was the heavily polluted steel town of Gary, Indiana.[17] Criticized for naming a town with such an enormous amount of pollution Green Town, Bradbury responded: "I was amused and somewhat astonished at a critic who wrote an article analyzing my novel, *Dandelion Wine*, plus the more realistic works of Sinclair Lewis, wondering how I could have been born and raised in Waukegan, which I renamed Green Town for my novel, and not noticed how ugly the harbor was and how depressing the coal docks and rail yards down below the town were. But, of course, I had noticed them and, genetic enchanter that I was, I was fascinated by their beauty."[18]

On one of my trips back home while my sister was sick, I drove down to the lakefront Bradbury wrote about and the place where my sister used to take me as a child. I stood on a pier next to the power plant. There was a tattered, faded sign stuck behind frozen glass—a warning not to eat the fish. Another sign told fisherman what to do with asbestos-coated pipe or other asbestos material should it wash up on-shore. There was a game warden and some bird-watchers on the pier just north of where my sister and I used to swim. I asked the warden for directions to the toxic-waste sites. He shouted out to me, his voice battling a whipping Lake Michigan wind: "Asbestos to the north; PCBs to the south." Once bounded on both sides by belching factories, the beach was now framed by abandoned buildings. Tall native prairie grasses grew between broken boards bent over by Lake Michigan winds. Bradbury was right. It was eerily beautiful.

CHAPTER THREE

Coho Capital of the World

꩜

W HETHER YOU ARE
fishing for them on boats with beers and friends or eating
them weekly at church-sponsored fundraisers, freshwater
fish in the towns bordering the Great Lakes are like pasta
in Italy—a signature dish, the centerpiece of a culture and
a catalyst that draws people together. On Lake Michigan,
the fish played another role too, one I learned about long
after I left home: the fish we ate as children created a tasty
and uninterrupted pathway from factory outflows to dinner
plates all along the shores of the lake—including the ones at
my house.

My father was a fisherman. He fished from the pier in
our hometown or out in the lake. We often ate his take for
dinner, and sometimes, when money was tight, we ate it for
breakfast too. In summer he stocked the freezer so we
would have a supply on hand when winter came. Where
once his catch might have been native whitefish, trout, and
perch, by the time I was growing up the lake's native stocks
had dwindled and certain species had all but disappeared.
As a result, my father sometimes brought home a fish for

dinner that the state had introduced into the lake in the 1960s, the coho salmon. The coho were brought in to restore the sport-fishing industry in what was by then a deeply troubled body of water.

The introduction of the coho was wildly successful. It drew anglers from around the Midwest to Waukegan and other ports and revitalized recreational fishing on the lake. But the fatty coho that was exciting to stalk and fun to catch also turned out to be a perfect repository for the PCB-laced fluid that the Outboard Marine Corporation factory contributed to the lake. By the time fishing bans were instituted in the 1970s, the coho were showing such high levels of toxins that the federal government eventually seized thousands of pounds of the fish, declaring it unfit to eat. It was a lake effect like no other, the result of a series of disastrous interactions between man and nature whose consequences are still felt today.

The first European explorers to see the Great Lakes called them the *mers douces*, or the sweet seas, but when I was growing up it was more common to call them dying or dead. Overfishing, intense shoreline development, the dumping of untreated sewage and industrial wastes into the lake, and the introduction of invasive aquatic species all contributed to destabilizing the ecology of the lakes and their fish populations.

The lake trout, for example, once a Lake Michigan staple, was all but wiped out by a combination of factors, including aggressive wounds from an invasive parasitic creature called the sea lamprey and the effects of industrial pollutants like PCBs that washed out of Waukegan's harbor. Research has shown that the high levels of pollution in the lake during the 1970s, particularly PCBs and dioxins, could single-handedly have set off an avalanche of unwelcome changes in fish populations, including the extirpation of the lake trout.[1]

In this destabilized environment, one small fish took hold: the alewife, a silvery fish that grows to about four to six inches long in the Great Lakes. Alewives are a saltwater fish native to the Atlantic coast, not the Great Lakes, and the tiny fish struggled mightily to survive in the freshwater of the lake. Rising and falling in great numbers, the alewife population would come to dominate only to die off in great waves and cover the lakeshores with their carcasses.

One fisherman reported seeing "miles of dead alewives floating in windrows three feet deep and three hundred yards wide."[2] Another outdoorsman recalled that the waves pushed the tiny dead fish into waist-high piles on the beach that could easily be smelled a mile away.[3] Still another homeowner remembered that it would take up to three hours to clear the small beachfront near their cabin of the dead, stinking fish. My sister and I used to throw the dead little fish at each other until their numbers or their smell drove us from the beach entirely.

I was eight years old in the summer of 1967 when a dramatic die-off sent massive numbers of dead alewives to shore. The decaying fish formed a stinking, sickening carpet on the beach—so thick that authorities had to use dump trucks to cart away mounds of the tiny dead fish. Even to a child, it was an unmistakable sign that the problems in the lake had reached crisis proportions.

Under pressure from homeowners, the tourism industry, and others to do something, Great Lakes fishing authorities hit upon a bold strategy: they introduced another new invasive species—a predator—to control the alewife population.

The fish they stocked—the coho salmon—was big and fun to catch, and it thrived on the alewife.

One million coho eggs arrived from Oregon in 1965, and the juvenile fish were raised in Michigan hatcheries. The first release came the following year in a "golden bucket ceremony" on the Platte River near Honor, Michigan.4 Naturalist Jerry Dennis, who grew up nearby, says the lakes came alive in 1967, the first year that the salmon reached maturity. They "grew at an unprecedented rate," he writes. "By August of 1967, people in aircraft saw schools of salmon three or four miles long swimming toward Platte Bay. The word spread. A kind of gold rush mentality prevailed."5

It is hard to overstate the craze that sport fishing brought to the lakes. People called it coho fever, and the local economy boomed overnight. Hotels were booked solid and fishing equipment sold out. People from as far away as Pennsylvania and Tennessee came to fish in the Great Lakes; some had never seen the lakes before, some had never fished before. The value of lake property along the "coho coast," where the fish ran, doubled. Boat ramps, a rarity on Lake Michigan before the arrival of the coho, sprang up overnight.6

Waukegan was eager to capitalize on this enthusiasm and started billing itself at the "Coho Capital of the World." The town began its own annual Coho Derby in 1968. Sponsored by Pepsi, the event drew fisherman from all over the country.7 Indeed, the excitement of catching the fish is hard to downplay. I remember the look in my father's eyes after he had come in from a day on the lake. The coho proved to be fish ecstasy for the men who sought sport fish. Jerry Dennis captures the thrill of it: "We were hooked more deeply than the fish we caught. We took salmon home and filleted them or cut them into steaks and ate them baked, grilled, broiled, and fried. What we couldn't eat we froze or canned or gave away to friends."[8] Everyone did the same, including my family, and they did it until the warnings started; some did it even *after* the warnings were posted.

Salmon are a fatty fish and that makes them tasty and hardy, but it also makes them excellent repositories for fat-soluble chemicals. PCBs are insoluble in water, but highly soluble in lipids, or fat. As a result, PCBs are gathered up in the food chain from the sediment where they had settled en masse. As larger fish eat smaller fish, the concentration of PCBs grows—a process scientists call biomagnification—so that fish at the top of the food chain can end up with an exposure many times greater than those at the bottom. For this reason, PCBs can make their way into the human body in concentrations dramatically higher than those that exist in the water.

It is helpful to look at the numbers to see how this works. Zooplankton and phytoplankton at the very bottom of the food chain in the Great Lakes had PCB concentrations of about 0.123 parts per million (ppm). The smelt that ate those organisms had typical concentrations about nine times higher, in the 1.04 ppm range. The trout that snacked on the smelt came in with concentrations of around 4.83 ppm. If you go higher still on the food chain and look at the eggs of herring gulls, they had PCB concentrations about 25 million times the concentration in the water. "The top predators at the end of a long food chain, such as lake trout, large salmon and fish-eating birds," warns the EPA, "may accumulate concentrations of a toxic chemical high enough to cause serious deformities or death even though the concentration of the chemicals in the open water is extremely low."[9]

By 1969, the top predators among the fish were so contaminated that the U.S. Food and Drug Administration (FDA) seized 34,000 pounds of Lake Michigan coho salmon, labeling it unfit for human consumption.[10] There were fish in the lake with whole-body PCB concentrations as high as 77 ppm—levels approximately 15 times the then-permissible 5 ppm.[11] The FDA's acceptable level today is 2 ppm, which puts the 1969 concentrations of PCBs at 38 times the acceptable level.[12] The eight Great Lakes states themselves now have a far more stringent standard of 0.05 ppm.[13] This means that the fish of my childhood contained 1,540 times the current limit.

The high levels of PCBs and other contaminants in the fish showed up in birds that ate the fish—most notably the cormorant—whose deformities and fertility problems were some of the first signs of trouble in the Great Lakes. Farmed mink that were fed the fish also developed serious fertility problems, and the kits that were born had high rates of mortality. These and other problems sent regulators and environmentalists searching for the sources of the problem. When it came to PCBs in particular, they found them in Waukegan.

"Animals that are exposed to high concentrations of pollutants often develop localized malignancies—tumors," writes the environmentalist William Ashworth. "Lakes, too, have localized malignancies from high concentrations of pollutants. These are the limnetic equivalents of tumors—or trouble spots, the places where the symptoms of poisoning first begin to show up. And along the Great Lakes, the worst of them all is at Waukegan, Illinois."[14]

As the extent of the pollution became clear, so did the full irony of the situation in Waukegan. The harbor that the people of Waukegan had dug a century before had lured industry and fishing interests with an unintended result: a company that made boat engines for fisherman had left the lake so polluted that it became impossible—or at least extremely dangerous—to eat the fish. Except we didn't know that at the time.

The pollution that had worked its way into the sediment would find its way into us through the fish, triggering a long cascade of events. And while the ramifications of the pollution were clear in animals, I was only beginning to understand the effects of the pollution on my sister and myself.

CHAPTER FOUR

The False Center of the Collage

⊚⟩

THE FIRST THING I SAW when I walked into my sister's memorial service was a collage of photographs, maybe forty of them on a large poster board—my sister at her high-school graduation, my sister as a bride, my sister as a new mother. I looked at one after another, cherishing her beauty, her gentleness. Then I saw it. The centerpiece of the collage was not a picture of my sister, but one of me alone. It was a picture of me at around eleven years old with my dog.

I stood staring at myself in a photo taken years before, with confusion and sadness rising in my chest. Someone had obviously mistaken me for my sister. That picture put me at the center of her life, her illness, and her death. It was a not so subtle reminder that our fates might be intertwined in ways I didn't want to think about.

The false center of that collage held a potent truth. A sibling's illness is not an isolated event. Every time a woman is diagnosed with breast or ovarian cancer, that diagnosis reverberates throughout the entire family. Sometimes subtle fear, sometimes a near panic, grips the whole family.

I can imagine a time when this would not have been true—a time before genetic testing, before invasive screening and imaging techniques, when a sister's disease did not cast such a long shadow. There must have been a time when a sister's cancer was her unique crisis. As her sibling, you would have taken care of her, or taken in her kids, or slipped in through the back door to bring a meal. But her diagnosis would have been hers alone. Not anymore. Today a sister's illness catapults you into the middle of the medical establishment as swiftly as it puts her into treatment.

My sister was diagnosed with ovarian cancer in April 1992 at the age of forty-one. I was thirty-two years old and an editor at the *Harvard Business Review*. She called me one day at work, and her small voice pressed through the phone: "I have ovarian cancer." And then with her next exhale: "You have to get tested." Like most women, my sister knew that ovarian cancer is a silent killer with few if any noticeable symptoms. She also knew that the disease sometimes runs in families.

I made the appointment to see a local gynecologist, if for nothing else than to assuage my sister. The doctor ordered the necessary blood tests, and I sat waiting to hear the results. My husband, Jon, arrived just in time to join me in the doctor's office. There is a blood marker for ovarian cancer, a cancer antigen called CA-125. Its presence at a certain level in your blood can mean that your body has mobilized against the disease, but the test is fraught with difficulties. Something as minor as a cold can trigger a false positive. Though the test is highly unreliable, it was the best diagnostic tool doctors had at the time.

"Your blood tests are fine," said the doctor. I thought about the relief I could bring my sister that night. I reveled in the fact that for me, at least for now, this cancer thing was not an issue. "But if I were you I would have a hysterectomy anyway," the doctor continued unexpectedly. "It is too dangerous," she said. "Ovarian cancer is too hard to detect, too hard to cure."

She told us that the strongest risk factor for ovarian cancer was having a family history of the disease and that the person at the highest risk for developing ovarian cancer was someone whose nearest relative with the disease was a sister.[1] That put me squarely in the high-risk category. Women in the general population with no affected relatives have a 1–2 percent chance of developing ovarian cancer. Women like myself, however, with a first-degree relative with the disease, have a 2–6 percent chance of developing the disease. The doctor repeated, "I would have a hysterectomy if I were you."

Astonished, we mentioned wanting children. The doctor pressed for details of our sex life—how often, during what times of my cycle. We had been married for five years and had been having unprotected sex for almost two. "Couples are considered infertile if they have been trying to have children for a year without success," she said flatly, looking at my husband and at me. We were both stunned silent.

I had known from my work as a journalist that some scientists were concerned that women who ate fish from Lake Michigan could develop fertility problems. A study would eventually be published in *Epidemiology* that correlated the amount of fish eaten and the amount of time it took women in the study to conceive.[2] The odds that a woman would become pregnant during a given menstrual cycle decreased in direct proportion to the amount of Great Lakes fish she had eaten.

Still, until that moment in the doctor's office I had never thought of myself as infertile, so I had never thought that my childhood diet of Lake Michigan fish might be playing a role in my ability to have children. The doctor, however, did not mince words. She thought we were infertile and she didn't much care why. She wanted us to get moving, to get to the fertility clinic and get started. She wanted me to have my children and then have my ovaries removed. She was certain I would need help getting pregnant. The first step was to shoot my uterus full of dye to see if my tubes were blocked. I made an appointment, then canceled it, and then went through with it.

I was fine as far as the tests could tell, well enough to go through the rigors of fertility treatment. Still, I hesitated. I distrusted the fertility drugs and I had heard that they sometimes swelled your ovaries to the size of small tomatoes during treatment. A widely debated and quite controversial study at the time reported a dramatic increase in ovarian cancer among women who had used fertility drugs.[3] Around the same time, a popular women's magazine editor who had been diagnosed with ovarian cancer wrote an article in which she persuasively argued that fertility drugs had played a role in her disease.[4]

Using my perch as an editor at the *Harvard Business Review*, I called specialists at Boston hospitals for advice. Everything I heard scared me: (1) not only was I at greater risk for ovarian cancer because of my sister's disease, I was also at greater risk for breast cancer; (2) the fact that I was having trouble becoming pregnant suggested I had undetected ovarian irregularities that put me at greater risk for ovarian cancer in the future; (3) not having had children earlier in life had increased my risk; (4) removing my ovaries would not guarantee that I would not get cancer in tissues similar in origin to ovarian tissues—such as the ones covering my abdominal organs.

Most of the doctors agreed that the suggestion of a hysterectomy was extreme, but certainly not unheard of. No one was sure about the link between the fertility drugs and cancer, but no one pooh-poohed it either. My husband, Jon, and I talked it over and decided that taking the drugs was not worth the risk. Besides, one potential side effect of the drugs was emotional instability. And I was already crying every day, sometimes for hours. I cried on the way to work, on the way home from work, and sometimes in the bathroom at work. Once I cried while swimming in the pool—my tears filling my goggles.

I cried for my sister. I cried because I didn't think I could have children. I cried because I was afraid that if I did have children I would die of ovarian cancer when they were little or that I would pass on this horrible disease to them, or both. I cried because I wanted children. Then I cried because I wanted children but didn't want my ovaries anymore. A hysterectomy would throw me into menopause, and that made me cry too.

So Jon and I frantically tried to have children without any high-tech assistance, squeezing sex in between his court appearances as a federal prosecutor and my frequent airplane departures for business or to see my sister. Where once our sex had been leisurely and loving, it now had to be carefully calibrated to coincide with my most fertile moments. I counted the days—days until I ovulated, days until I should have my period. Then when my period came, I started counting all over again. Meanwhile, my sister counted her own days—a year maybe, or two, max—that's what she had been told. Another drug might work for her unless it became too toxic. A bone-marrow transplant might work but could be fatal. And so went the slow calculation of life and death. Until it happened.

Sometime after my sister's bone-marrow transplant but before the final fatal recurrence of her cancer, I became pregnant. I flew from Boston to her house just west of Waukegan to tell her in her backyard. As I told her, tears pooled at the edge of her eyes, massing where her eyelashes would have been if they had not been vaporized by chemotherapy, and then they ran down her face in jagged little rivers.

"I prayed for this," she said.

I was able to visit my sister a few more times before my baby was born. I teased her about her wig, called her Church Lady after the then-popular *Saturday Night Live* character. We went shopping for clothes as we always had. We did it methodically, continually honing our skills in practice runs while we circled our prey. But as the seasons changed, the reality of her disease took hold. She refused to buy clothes for the winter, arguing forcefully that she might not need them.

I remember my sister handing me a small picture in a frame. In the picture she wears a white lace minidress. Her long legs are bent seductively at the knee. Her hair is swept off her neck in a chignon. I am standing next to her in a straight yellow chiffon dress with a high, ruffled collar—my hair hangs sloppily over one eye. She has her hand on my shoulder in true big-sister style. Remember us like this, she told me. And I do.

They stopped her chemotherapy on my due date, February 15, 1995. She had made it just far enough, and there was nothing more to do but wait—she for death and me for the birth of my child.

I would see her one more time. Three weeks after Jacob was born, I hobbled through O'Hare Airport with him, still recovering from his cesarean birth. Sue was thin and propped up on her couch at home. I laid my son on her chest as she lay dying. His lips turned into a little smile and he fell fast asleep. Her tears dripped on his head, a baptism that brought him into the cycle of living and dying. He slept peacefully until it was time to go. She handed him back to me and said, "He is the future." She died when Jacob was eight weeks old.

CHAPTER FIVE

Lake Michigan Legacy

ⵣ

MY SON MIGHT BE THE future, as my sister told me on her deathbed, but even then I feared he would be marked indelibly by my past. Chemicals like those in the lake at the foot of my hometown are known to persist for decades in the environment and in the human body, and they can be transferred to a fetus across the placenta and to an infant in breast milk. Exposures in infancy and in utero are particularly dangerous to children. Scientists believe that minute early exposures to toxins may set the stage for cancers such as breast and prostate to develop later in life.

Toxic interferences in brain development, in addition, can cause long-term deficits. A study published in the *New England Journal of Medicine* in 1996 followed 212 children from infancy to age eleven whose mothers had eaten Lake Michigan fish contaminated with PCBs. The researchers found lower than average IQ scores, poor reading skills, memory problems, and attention deficits in the children—effects that persisted into late childhood.[1] More recently, Harvard researchers drew attention to 202 chemicals—

including PCBs—that can damage the human brain. These chemicals, the authors contended, are creating a "silent pandemic" that is wreaking havoc with our children's ability to learn. The effects cited included shortened attention spans, slowed motor coordination, and heightened aggressiveness.[2]

As I tried to learn more about Waukegan's pollution and to fulfill my promise to my sister to write about it, each fact I learned, each study I read, seemed only to expand my questions and concerns. First I was motivated by my sister's cancer, then by my infertility, and finally by my very real concern about my son. So in the years after Jacob was born, I once again started to learn about the chemicals of my childhood.

PCBs were first synthesized in 1881 by German chemists searching for dyes. PCBs failed as dyes and their use was limited until scientists discovered that their heat-resistant properties made them ideal for use as lubricants and as insulation in industrial machinery and electrical equipment.[3] PCBs were first manufactured commercially in the United States in 1929 by Swann Chemical and later by Monsanto.[4] Colorless, odorless, and tasteless, PCBs do not burn, conduct electricity, or change their behavior in response to alterations in pH. One writer called them "the mules of the chemical world."[5]

The first indication that the chemicals were dangerous to human health came in the mid-1930s, when three employees at a Halowax Corporation factory in New York City fell sick after being exposed to them. The workers were covered with an aggravated skin rash called chloracne—an acute complication resulting from heavy exposure to PCBs or dioxins. When two of the workers subsequently died, autopsies revealed severe liver damage. A Harvard researcher was called in to investigate, and he discovered that test rats, after repeated dosing with PCBs, also developed liver damage.

The researcher subsequently presented his findings to Monsanto and to the owners of the plant where the men were exposed. "These experiments leave no doubt as to the possibility of systemic effects" from the chemicals, he said.[6] His report was ultimately published in a scholarly journal, but little attention was paid to it. As a result, concerns about PCBs—to the extent that they were acknowledged at all— would remain largely an issue for individual manufacturers and their employees until widespread persistence of PCBs in the environment was discovered in the late 1960s.

The 1962 publication of Rachel Carson's landmark book *Silent Spring*, and its serialization in the *New Yorker*, brought attention to an enormous increase in the number of synthetic chemicals (of which PCBs are one type) available for use in post–Word War II homes, industry, and agriculture. "The chemicals to which life is asked to make its adjustment are no longer merely the calcium and silica and copper and all the rest of the minerals washed out of the rocks and carried in rivers to the sea," wrote Carson. "They are the synthetic creations of man's inventive mind, brewed in his laboratories, and having no counterparts in nature."[7]

Carson most famously campaigned against the pesticide DDT and its devastating effects on wildlife. Her book and the popular outcry it created sent waves of scientists searching for remnants of the pesticide in birds worldwide. One of those was the Swedish chemist Søren Jensen. Searching for DDT in eagles and other species near his homeland, Jensen found a mystery chemical that was a close chemical cousin of DDT. He would later name it a PCB, after its chemical structure, and marvel when he found it in samples almost everywhere he looked—even in hair samples from his wife and children.

There are 209 varieties of PCBs. Each has a somewhat different chemical structure, but common to all are two hexagon-shaped benzene rings with hydrogen and chlorine atoms attached.[8] The two rings are attached by a carbon-to-carbon bond, so diagrammatically they look like a pair of eyeglasses or two bicycle wheels attached by a thin strip.[9]

Because each PCB variety bears its own signature design, the chemicals can often be traced to their source—they can be fingerprinted, so to speak. Working with a German chemist, Jensen correctly identified PCBs as chemicals widely used in modern manufacturing, and by fingerprinting their chemical structure he was eventually able to trace them to their source.[10] Jensen's work, published in the *New Scientist* in 1966, set off a tidal wave of study on the chemicals, their uses, and their persistence in birds, animals, and humans that continues today.

In the Great Lakes region, naturalists and birders were the first to bring the dangers of these chemicals to the public's attention. Reports of a decline in the population of bald eagles and deformities in the chicks of double-crested cormorants began to surface in the 1960s and 1970s. Adding to the alarm were reports of birds born with crossed bills that made it impossible for them to eat, or birds born with stomachs outside their bodies and with shortened appendages, missing eyes or brains.[11]

Birth defects in double-crested cormorants, such as the crossed bill, were 42 percent more likely in the Great Lakes area than in cormorant colonies outside elsewhere. Fish, especially bottom-feeders such as catfish and carp, also began to show effects, including tumors and liver cancers.[12] And, as mentioned earlier, minks fed Great Lakes fish suffered serious bouts of infertility.[13]

But it took a tragic accident in the Japanese city of Kitakyushu to reveal the powerfully poisonous effects of PCBs. In 1968, on the northern tip of the island of Kyushu, one thousand people were affected when rice oil inadvertently became infused with PCBs during manufacturing. Five people died and residents reported a long list of ailments that included a ravaging form of acne, jaundice, nausea, vomiting, and abdominal cramps.[14] This incident gave rise to a new word in the Japanese language, *yusho*, or Japanese rice-oil disease.[15] Japan promptly banned the chemicals, and a similar ban would follow in the United States in 1976.[16]

Evidence from the Japanese tragedy led to international concerns about PCBs. Monsanto was the sole producer in North America and made the chemicals in vast quantities.[17] Their uses were multiple. PCBs were added to pesticides to make them flow more easily from planes that were aerating crops, for example.[18] Another manufacturer added them to chewing gum, while farmers added them to the paint used inside grain silos. And not far from the house in which I grew up, PCB-laced fluid was used to keep down the dirt on a local track.

The chemical was virtually everywhere. Between 1969 and 1971, news reports listed nine major PCB contaminations of food, from cereal to chickens. In one well-publicized instance, 140,000 tainted chickens had to be destroyed before they were made into chicken soup.[19] By 1972, PCBs had been found in every major river in the United States and in all the Great Lakes.[20]

One of the largest point sources of PCB pollution in the Great Lakes during the 1960s and 1970s was located in my hometown. The Outboard Marine Corporation used the chemicals voluminously in the manufacture of boat motors marketed under the brand names Evinrude and Johnson, the names of two early owners of the company.[21] In fact, it was Ole Evinrude, a Milwaukee engineer, who made the first detachable boat motor in 1908. The outboards began as a novelty. But by the mid-1920s, detachable motors became popular—even necessary—for fisherman and those who lived near the water. In 1927, the growing company moved to Waukegan for the town's lakeside location and easy railroad access.

By 1952, Outboard Marine had made one million motors on the shores of Lake Michigan. The following year the company completed construction of a new die-casting building that was called the "finest installation of its kind in the world."[22] The company needed the additional space to build the Johnson Sea Horse, a model that in a single year would outsell every other outboard motor ever made.[23] "It's sensational!" actor Gary Cooper jauntily said in company advertising. Amazing too was the Waukegan plant's production record in manufacturing: one million motors made in just five years.

By the late 1960s, the company operated 127 die-casting machines, each weighing between 600 and 1,600 tons, running day and night in a lakefront plant that covered twenty-three acres.[24] Given the enormous mold-clamping forces—sometimes more than 2,000 tons per square inch—and the high pressure and heat of the molten metal needed to form the motor parts, the mechanism of each die-casting machine required a durable hydraulic fluid in large quantity that would allow it to produce, withstand, and transmit enormous forces and not catch fire or explode.[25]

A few years earlier, in 1954, the company began purchasing the PCB-laden hydraulic fluid called Pydraul from Monsanto. Over the next seventeen years—until Monsanto stopped selling the fluid for use in open systems such as the one in Waukegan—Outboard Marine bought between 10 and 11 million pounds of Pydraul. Roughly 10 percent of that amount would come to rest on the lake bed in the harbor.

Unfortunately, the same chemical stability that made the fluid suitable for industrial use also made its toxicity persistent in the environment. Documents from one of the first lawsuits concerning the pollution state the facts succinctly: "In 1976 the government determined that an estimated 1.1 million pounds of PCBs rested on the bed of the harbor."[26] Many more pounds made their way to landfills, and some went into the air via burning. The numbers for water, land, and air pollution are staggering. Here is how it stacks up.

In the Water

Die-casting machines produce an enormous amount of heat as they operate. At Outboard Marine, large quantities of metalworking fluids were poured onto the hot metal of the machines and allowed to run off into troughs along the factory floor. Under the immense pressures required for casting, hydraulic fluids containing PCBs also leaked into the cooling system, and used cooling water containing PCBs was sent back to the lake through a ditch stretching to the harbor.

It is likely that some direct dumping occurred as well. Hydraulic fluids and metalworking fluids, like car-engine oil and brake fluid, need to be changed at regular intervals and the old fluids disposed of. At least one memo from plant management suggests that the 37,000-gallon holding tanks of hydraulic fluid associated with each machine were changed twice a year.[27] It is likely that some, if not all, of that used fluid was dumped into the harbor. Indeed, it is hard to imagine that the high concentrations of PCBs in the harbor could have been achieved without some direct dumping of fluids. An operator of a marina business adjacent to Outboard Marine, for example, reported in sworn depositions that he had to wipe boats clean of oil from the slicks created daily by the motor manufacturing company.[28]

The following 1974 letter from a plant engineer to management, written well after the danger from PCBs was established, explains what had likely been going on for almost twenty years:

> Individuals at both plants are dumping five-gallon containers of soluble oil directly into storm sewer floor drains. To cite specific examples, at Plant #1 last Monday and Thursday, September 23 and 26 at approximately 8:00 AM, soluble oil was discharged into the harbor from Plant #1. This has been a regular occurrence every four and five days since the last plant shutdown. The soluble oil enters the harbor each time between 8:00 AM and 8:15 AM which indicates a pattern that a person is dumping the oil into a floor drain at approximately 7:15 AM. . . . A week ago Monday night, September 2, a vast quantity of soluble oil was discharged into the north ditch.[29]

By the time the PCB problem was isolated in January 1976, the Illinois Environmental Protection Agency believed that Outboard Marine was delivering approximately nine to ten pounds of PCBs to the harbor each day.[30] The PCB content of the sludge at the bottom of the harbor ranged from 240,000 to 500,000 parts per million depending on when and where the sample was taken.[31] That means that either one in two or one in four grains of sand or silt at the bottom of the harbor was not actually sand or silt, but was a PCB instead. To grasp the magnitude of the pollution, compare these numbers to the current acceptable limit for sediment set by the EPA of 0.2 parts per million. That amounts to pollution in the harbor that is *one to two million times* currently acceptable levels.

In this context it is worth remembering the history of the harbor. It is not a natural inlet, but is rather a "slack harbor," meaning that there is no river or stream that might carry sediments away from the harbor. To keep it navigable, the harbor needed to be dredged to a depth of twenty-three feet as mandated by the U.S. Army Corps of Engineers.[32] The harbor was dredged yearly until the massive amounts of PCB pollution were officially "discovered" in 1976. Thereafter, dredging was discontinued because it can stir up so much toxic sentiment. Some of the dredged material was dumped onto Outboard Marine's property, and some was dragged two thousand feet south of the harbor and deposited in open water where engineers built a "sand mountain."[33] Other reports locate the dredged materials out farther—about three miles—in deep water.[34] As a result of these dredging activities, polluted sediment similar to the type found in the harbor has been discovered as far as six miles out into the lake.[35]

Contaminated sediment suspended in the lake's water may also have entered Waukegan's drinking water. The town's emergency water intake sits near the original source of pollution in the harbor, and the main water intake lies 6,244 feet out into the lake.[36] At least once, in 1988, harbor water entered the town's drinking water intake. Whether that happened consistently—especially in the days before the extent of the pollution was understood—is an open question.[37]

On Land

A sizable amount of the PCB-laden fluids used by Outboard Marine also dripped onto the factory floor, where it was cleaned up using sawdust or a kitty-litter-like substance. The oil-infused material was put into barrels and carted away by private companies. Outboard Marine's own documents show that between 1959 and 1971 somewhere between five and seven million pounds of contaminated waste was carted off.

In an unhappy coincidence, the company that had the contract to remove wastes from the plant also had the contract to run the city landfill. The landfill was less than a mile from our house, abutted the farm where our family bought vegetables, and was also neighbor to the apartment building where my brother once lived. In a story that would repeat itself again and again across the country, the industrial waste that fell on the shop floor ended up in an unlined landfill that would, tragically and predictably, leak.

The local newspaper, the *Waukegan News-Sun*, described the leaking landfill and its stinking leachate in 1972.

It isn't difficult to find—just follow your nose. [Yeoman Creek] flows north to south along the west edge of the old dump. Two dozen small streams of foul-smelling, rusty-colored liquid trickle from the dump directly into the creek. Called leachate, the liquid is decomposed garbage washed out of the dump by rainfall. It turns Yeoman Creek into an ugly, red-colored sewage drain. The creek absorbs the stinking ooze as it flows along the dump and carries it downstream under Glen Flora Avenue into Yeoman Park, Powell Park and Washington Park where hundreds of Waukegan children will play this summer. Eventually the ooze is washed out into Lake Michigan.[38]

The Yeoman Creek landfill opened when the town's previous landfill, Edwards Field, which operated from 1958 to 1963, became full. The two adjacent sites occupy about seventy acres and are separated only by a set of high-tension power lines. After Yeoman Creek opened, Edwards Field was reclaimed as a recreational area. To celebrate, Mayor Sabonjian threw a party for town residents complete with tea and crumpets, a brass band, and an exhibition baseball game.[39] The Little League ball fields remained in use until well after the discovery that they were built on an oozing mess of PCBs and other chemicals, including benzene, trichloroethylene, arsenic, lead, phthalates, and cyanide.[40]

Apartments, businesses, a restaurant, and a nursing home where my grandmother lived surrounded the conjoined landfills. In 1985, a small fire broke out in the nursing home and PCBs were discovered in the building's basement sump pump—presumably having come up through the groundwater.

In the Air

Until recently, scientists did not view airborne PCBs as a critical exposure pathway, but that is beginning to change. "We have very strong evidence that inhalation is an important route of exposure that has not been appreciated," says David Carpenter, director of the Institute for Health and the Environment in Albany, New York.[41]

Outboard Marine had its own smelting operation, and scrap aluminum parts were melted there to be used again. The parts were often covered with hydraulic and metalworking fluids, and when the smelting took place PCBs were released as a vapor. The company estimates that in a two-year period they released between 300,000 and 434,000 pounds of PCBs into the air.[42]

Although Outboard Marine garnered the most publicity and the most regulatory and legal action for the pollution it generated, it was not alone. Many factories along the lake spewed chemicals into the air or water or dumped them on land, all of which could potentially lead to adverse health effects for area residents and wildlife. One plant used asbestos; a coal-tar plant released polyaromatic hydrocarbons; and a coal-fired power plant—called one of the dirtiest in the country—spewed mercury.

Land, lake, air: it all adds up to an enormous amount of pollution. So much that it is hard to imagine anyone dumping or leaking or spouting that much of any pollutant—in this case, PCBs—for that many years. Nefarious? In some instances, maybe. But there are two important things to consider when looking at the behavior of Outboard Marine and the other factories along the lake.

The first is that Outboard Marine's manufacturing

processes were in some respects standard operating procedure for their time. One consultant called the plant "immac-
ulate and well-organized" and ranked the company's
operations on a par with those of the German engineering
shop of Volkswagen.[43] In manufacturing and engineering in
the 1960s and 1970s, there was no higher compliment. It was
a time when many people did not consider the environmental effects of what they were doing or what might happen
when chemicals used in production combined with those
used in water treatment or waste disposal. In *The Road to
Love Canal*, Craig Colten and Peter Skinner report that in
the twenty-year period from about 1950 to 1970, 1,605
chemical plants acknowledged discarding approximately
762 million tons of waste. "By far," they write, "the most
common methods of disposal were landfills, pits, ponds, or
lagoons."[44]

The Waukegan story, then, while horrific in its own way,
is not unique. It is a story that has unfolded over and over
again across the American landscape. And even if Waukegan
officials had been more aware of the dangers, they still
might have chosen to look the other way. After the extent of
the pollution was well known and the dangers of the chemicals were well established, Mayor Sabonjian continued to
assert that there was "no proof that PCBs were harmful" and
that he had "never yet heard of anyone being injured by
PCBs from Waukegan Harbor."[45] If the mayor's message
was "commerce at all costs," it was because it was both a
profitable and politically popular message. In 1968 alone,
Outboard Marine paid wages of $23 million dollars—that's
around $150 million in today's dollars.

The second thing to remember when trying to understand the actions of Outboard Marine and other polluting

companies is that the vastness of the lakes has always fostered an erroneous impression that they can absorb an unending amount of waste.[46] In fact, just the opposite is true. Toxins that are spewed into the lake stay there. It takes a hundred years for the water in Lake Michigan to "turn over" and be replaced through accumulation of rainwater and the natural flows from its watershed. As a result, the concentrations of chemicals grow steadily rather than being diluted.

For those who looked carefully, Lake Michigan became an early warning system about the hazards of chemical pollution, not just for humans but for other life in the region too. "By the 1970s the levels of persistent toxic chemicals in the water itself grew alarmingly high," noted a Conservation Foundation report, *Great Lakes, Great Legacy*. "Waterfowl populations, fish, and wildlife dependent on the aquatic ecosystem were found laced with toxic contaminants, deformed, and dying."[47]

As the awareness of the problems with the lake grew, so did the consensus that something had to be done to protect one of the world's largest supplies of freshwater and the health of the people who lived along its shores. Among other government initiatives at the time, in 1975 the U.S. Environmental Protection Agency convened a national conference on PCBs to present relevant data on the persistence and toxicity of the chemicals. Regulation soon followed: PCBs were banned in 1976, except for limited uses. At the same time, the EPA was charged with regulating the disposal of existing PCBs.

In February of the same year, the U.S. EPA and the Illinois EPA issued an administrative enforcement order demanding the elimination of PCB discharges from Outboard

Marine outfalls within thirty days. Two years later, in 1978, as part of a new Great Lakes Water Quality Agreement with Canada, the two countries agreed to a "zero discharge" standard for the Great Lakes. That same year the U.S. EPA filed its first lawsuit against Outboard Marine and the manufacturer of Pydraul, Monsanto, for unauthorized dumping. Indeed, the Waukegan Outboard Marine site is now known not simply for the vast amount of pollution it generated, but also for the long and ugly legal battles associated with it.

For over a decade, Outboard Marine denied federal investigators access to their property while their lawyers battled attorneys from the U.S. EPA all the way to the Supreme Court. The EPA fought bitterly for access to the polluted property.[48] In 1980, Congress passed the Comprehensive Environmental Response, Compensation, and Liability Act (CERCLA), which created the Superfund and gave regulators increased power and authority over sites such as Outboard Marine's.

Unfortunately for those who sought to protect the environment through regulatory means, Ronald Reagan was elected president in 1981 on a probusiness, antiregulation platform that set the stage for massive rollbacks in environmental enforcement. As a young journalist at the time, I experienced the dramatic sea change from the Carter administration's attention to public health and safety to the Reagan administration's desire to allow businesses to operate unfettered.

Reagan appointed Anne Gorsuch to head the EPA. A former Mountain Bell Telephone attorney, Gorsuch had been a conservative state senator from Colorado who had once supported the use of a federally banned chemical to kill coyotes.[49] As her chief of staff, Gorsuch chose someone from the asbestos industry, and to head the agency's air-pollution effort she chose a woman who had lobbied for a paper company. To head the Superfund program, Gorsuch appointed a woman who had worked in public relations for a large aerospace concern, with its own environmental problems related to a Superfund site. Her name was Rita Lavelle.

Gorsuch's first step was to dismantle the EPA's enforcement division, essentially gutting the Superfund legislation. Legislators, realizing that Gorsuch and Lavelle were out to dismantle the EPA, demanded materials related to the running of the agency, particularly the Superfund program. Gorsuch, with the backing of the White House, refused to hand over the documents, and as a result she became the first cabinet official in U.S. history to be cited for contempt of Congress.[50] Lavelle would later serve time in jail for lying to Congress.

The Waukegan Outboard Marine site landed in the midst of the scandal when it was revealed that Lavelle had tried to cut a backdoor deal more favorable to the company than the one officially put forth by her agency—a common practice at the time. "It was a well-known fact that if a company didn't like what it was getting in negotiations with agency lawyers, it could go to the assistant administrator, the deputy administrator, or to Gorsuch's office," said one U.S. Department of Justice official. "They could just go all the way up the ladder to get what they wanted."[51]

Although the scandal in Washington probably delayed a cleanup in Waukegan, it did not derail it. In 1986, a revised Superfund law went into effect that clearly favored regulators, and years of battling over access to the Outboard Marine property ended. At that point, negotiations began in earnest to settle the suits, and plans for the cleanup began.

Commenting on the case many years later, a writer for the *Chicago Tribune* said, "The agency took a difficult case and made it a milestone that could make other pollution disputes easier to resolve."[52]

A final consent decree was signed with Outboard Marine in 1988. Contaminated sediment from the harbor was placed in containment cells during a $21 million cleanup that was paid for by the company. An embattled Outboard Marine closed its plant in 1998, three years after my sister died. In December 2000, the company went bankrupt and abandoned its buildings on the lakefront. Six years later, the town began tearing down some of the company's vacated buildings.[53]

Unfortunately, the legacy remains. Given the area's long history of industrial use, cleaning it up has been like taking a course in toxic archaeology. Each layer reveals another set of contaminants. "Every time we clean something up," says Evan Craig of the Sierra Club, "we find something else."[54] Federal EPA officials say that certain groundwater tests underneath some of the buildings near the harbor have turned up water that is literally black.

Some areas that did not qualify for federally funded restitution were designated Illinois EPA sites and left to wait their turn for cleanup. Two of these sites were so polluted that the gases they emitted ignited and the buildings either exploded or burned—including a paint factory and a tannery. The tar pits near the harbor were so degraded that six great blue herons that landed on them sank into the toxic muck and died.[55]

Only a fraction of the PCBs have ever been found. Much may have been dispersed through the food chain or may still be in the lake. As one official is fond of saying, "The plant used 11 million pounds of PCBs, we have found about 1 million pounds. So where's the other 10 million pounds?"[56]

Such a question may sound rhetorical. But for me and many, many others, it is personal as well. Biologically potent amounts of PCBs are likely to continue to show up in Great Lakes fish and in the people who eat them for a very long time. My sister and I ate a good deal of that fish, and I needed to know what effect those chemicals might have on me. Moreover, I was beginning to understand that my son, too, could possibly suffer the effects of those fish if they had left me with a chemical body burden that could cross into my womb and seep out through my breast milk. I may have been a fact-crazed girl with lots of facts, but surprisingly these facts, this story, left me with more questions than answers.

CHAPTER SIX

A Marked Woman

As the extent of the pollution in the Great Lakes became clear, a silent truth rolled over the water like a gathering storm: the lakes had become one large, uncontrolled experiment testing the effects of dioxins, PCBs, and other synthetic chemicals in wildlife and humans alike. Waukegan, despite its dramatic pollution, was just one of forty-three areas of concern designated by U.S. and Canadian officials. The scene that played out in my hometown was repeated again and again around the lakes. Toxicologists, developmental biologists, wildlife specialists, and birders were all reporting changes in wildlife. The lake effect was real, and it was creating a storm like no other.

The fish and the birds showed perhaps the most dramatic effects from the chemicals. Bottom-feeders such as catfish that dug in contaminated sediment near outflow pipes developed large, bulbous tumors near their mouths, on the side of their heads, or behind their eyes. Some young fish were seen swimming upside down in highly polluted waters. Other fish had liver tumors. Birds displayed mating irregularities and birth defects.

Theo Colborn watched the data accumulate during the 1980s. It wasn't until her children were grown and she turned fifty that this rural Colorado pharmacist was able to follow her dream and study zoology. With a newly minted PhD, she landed a job at the Conservation Foundation in Washington, DC, and began working on a Great Lakes project.

Colborn collected hundreds of studies on diverse birds, fish, and wildlife. Sorting through boxes and boxes of reports documenting changes in fish, birds, and other wildlife thought to have been caused by widespread toxic contamination, Colborn decided to enter her findings on a large spreadsheet. She put all of the wildlife along one axis and listed their defects, deformities, and behavioral changes along another. She soon saw a pattern emerging. The top predators showed more effects than other wildlife. That made sense, since the chemicals were known to bioaccumulate, concentrating in larger and larger amounts as they traveled up the food chain. Colborn's spreadsheet revealed another interesting finding too: the chemicals in the lakes were affecting organs like the thyroid, the ovaries, the mammary glands, and the pancreas—all endocrine glands that secrete hormones.

Colborn's work was first published in 1990 in the groundbreaking book *Great Lakes, Great Legacy*, but that was just the beginning. Soon, reports from other highly polluted areas revealed the effects synthetic chemicals might be having on animals. Baby alligators in a Florida lake contaminated by a chemical company's DDT spill developed penises only half normal size, a condition the media dubbed "teeny weenies." These animals looked like females and had elevated levels of estrogen in their blood. The offspring of frogs, turtles, and other wildlife exposed to pesticides, herbicides, and industrial discharges also showed significant changes in sex characteristics and hormone levels. The evidence eventually included seventy studies that showed effects of synthetic chemicals and pesticides across eight taxa—fish, mammals, birds, reptiles, sea urchins (echinoderms), worms, mollusks, and zooplankton. The media soon dubbed the chemicals "gender benders."[1]

As reports of similar problems began to come in from distant parts of the country and from all over the world, the trickle of studies became a flood, and a group of scientists decided to gather in 1991 to share their work. Appropriately enough, the group met at the Wingspread conference center in Racine, Wisconsin, just a few miles north of Waukegan. The result was the now well-accepted theory and landmark statement that chemical contaminants, from DDT to PCBs, disrupt the endocrine system of wildlife and are particularly deleterious to their offspring. Colborn remembers the meeting at which this idea first crystallized. "It was an epiphany," she says.[2] The epiphany, however, was incomplete. Hanging in the air was the unanswered question: if these endocrine-disrupting chemicals had this effect on wildlife, what kind of effect were they having on humans?

This was the question I was struggling with almost ten years after the emergence of the endocrine-disruption theory. It was 2000, I was forty years old and living in Boston with my husband and then five-year-old son, who blessedly showed no development delays or other symptoms associated with PCBs or other synthetic chemical toxicity.

I had not been able to have a second child, though. I continued to follow news reports on the effects of the chemicals in the Great Lakes, and my toxic exposure as a young girl weighed heavily on my mind. My husband and I tried intrauterine insemination without the drugs that had at one time been thought to promote ovarian cancer. Drive-by insemination, we used to call it. My husband would get up early, go to the clinic and make his "deposit" in a small plastic cup, and head to work. I would get my son up, drop him off at day care, and drive to the clinic where I would be inseminated. At no time during the process did we see each other. We did this five or six times, fighting traffic to get to the clinic and then fighting traffic to get into work. No luck.

Short of using ovary-stimulating treatments, there was not much the fertility doctors could do for us. They called it unexplained infertility. But I knew a few things about the pollution I had been exposed to back home. In the car on the way to the fertility clinic, my mind would drift back to the fish in Lake Michigan. I remembered that minks fed on fat-rich coho had fertility problems, one of the first indications that the chemicals in the lake were dangerous, and I knew that this could also affect women who ate the salmon. I also knew from earlier research I had read that couples with the greatest difficulty conceiving were those who had eaten the most fish from the Great Lakes.[3]

My promise to my sister and my fears about the chemicals in the lake had lingered in my mind for years; now my fertility difficulties gave me additional incentive to delve deeper into the problems associated with the lake. And so with guilt, fear, and morbid fascination as my motivators, I renewed my efforts to write the account I had promised my sister. I had a more immediate reason as well. If, as I suspected, the chemicals had made it impossible for me to have a second child, I needed to know what other effects my earlier exposures might be having on my health. Knowledge for knowledge's sake was all well and good, but I wanted to know more about how these chemicals might be affecting my body.

My first step was to see my sister's oncologist and obtain her health records, not only to learn more about her condition, but to try to make sense of my own risks and to make my own choices. If you are a woman, it turns out that your health history starts with your sister.

Even to get an appointment with my sister's oncologist in Chicago, I had to speak first with his assistant, who contacted the office manager, who checked with my insurance company. Only when the doctor's office was sure that I was not trying to sue or was not about to come apart emotionally were they willing to make the appointment.

Arming myself against what I knew would be a difficult trip, I took what can only be called defensive action. I bought a first-class ticket, a first-rate cashmere wrap, and reserved a car for the forty-five-minute drive from O'Hare.

I found the doctor's office in a nondescript building off the Illinois toll road. In his waiting room, a woman sat transfixed before a fish tank, practicing some kind of relaxation ritual before her appointment. She looked worried, and why not? Most people do not casually visit oncologists.

I picked up a *People* magazine and sat toward the back of the room. A Muzak version of "Wipe Out," a drum solo from the 1960s, was on the radio. For a brief moment I looked around to see if anyone else found this bizarre, but then I realized that I was the last living female member of my family. "Wipe Out" started to seem appropriate, festive even. I began tapping my foot to the beat, and then the nurse called my name.

The doctor, a tall, lanky man, ushered me in. After some

preliminaries, he told me what I already knew. My sister had lots of spunk. She asked a lot of questions. She wasn't—in his words—going to let anyone get away with anything. Then he laid out the facts.

My sister died of clear-cell ovarian adenocarcinoma in 1995 at the age of forty-four. Ovarian cancer is among the most deadly forms of cancer. Roughly twenty-five thousand cases are diagnosed each year, and about half of these result in death. Ovarian cancers are often diagnosed only at an advanced stage, which accounts for their high mortality rates. My sister's cancer was no exception. When it was found in 1992, it had spread beyond her ovaries to surrounding tissue. Despite aggressive chemotherapy and a bone-marrow transplant, Sue died just three years after she was diagnosed.

As I stood up to leave, the doctor handed me Sue's medical records and some pages from a book he had copied for me, outlining my own risk of developing ovarian cancer. "For women with a first-degree relative with ovarian cancer," the pages read, "such as a sister or mother, the lifetime chance to develop the disease is estimated at about 2 to 6 percent. Roughly double that of the general population."

Before I left for the airport, I stopped to buy flowers for the cemetery. The woman at the flower shop did not want the roses to die, and she wrapped them tight. I could not tell her that I would lay them on a frozen grave. We must presume life, I suppose, although as a preschooler my son used to say in his straightforward, chirpy way after stomping in from the backyard, "Mama, I need something to grave." I could barely resist saying, "Third cabinet from the left, that's where Mama always keeps the cadavers."

Jacob's preschool class had buried a much-loved pet, and

he had been taken with the beauty of the ritual—the quiet space, the sanctity of it all. The challenge, of course, is to make death a part of living. "Everything dies," I used to tell him. "Your sister died," he would repeat to me in his mantra-like way. "Yes," I would say and squeeze him hard, kissing him all over. "Mama!" he would squeal and wiggle away.

Back in Boston, with my sister's medical records, I finally registered at a large cancer center as a high-risk patient. Jon and I had abandoned efforts to have a second child, and I was now focused on the long-term health consequences of the chemicals.

There are three things that are striking about cancer hospitals. First, they always have enormous fish tanks full of multicolored, frisky fish. They are never floating sideways close to the top and near death. They are happy, energetic, cheerful fish. Second, there is always a lot of food around, usually junk food. On the day I arrived for the first time, it was donuts in great quantity. The third thing is related to the first two. There is always a long wait during which you are supposed to watch the fish (calming, pleasing) and eat the free donuts (strangely satisfying).

The first person I was registered to see was a geneticist, a brown-haired young woman whose perfectly coordinated outfit suggested a perfect academic transcript to match. Though I had my sister's medical records with me and a detailed family history, she offered little insight. There was not enough disease in my family for there to be a simple, straightforward genetic cause for my sister's disease.

All cancers are genetic in some form, since what drives cancer, scientists believe, is something in the genetic coding of a cell that causes it to reproduce in a crazy, unstoppable way. Cancer, however, is not usually considered a disease that is strictly or inevitably passed down in the genes you receive from your parents. Despite the fact that cancer is a genetic disease at the cellular level, as a general rule, it is not a disease with a major inherited component. Doctors at the hospital told me that only a small percentage of cancers, 5–10 percent, are strongly inherited.[4] So if you have a gene such as BRCA, you would be more likely to develop breast or ovarian cancer than the general population. But having the marker for that gene doesn't mean that you will definitely develop the disease.

In my case, my scant family history made it extremely unlikely that there was a strong inherited genetic link for my sister's disease. The letter they sent from the hospital made this clear: "Cancer is a common disease," it read, "and all of us start with about a 30% (1 in 3) chance of developing some type of cancer over the course of our lives. Women have a 1 in 9 (11%) chance of developing breast cancer and a 1 in 70 (1–2%) chance of developing ovarian cancer over the course of a lifetime."[5]

I might have stopped my searching and worry when I received this letter. I could easily have decided that because I didn't carry the BRCA gene, the best-known genetic marker for ovarian cancer, I had little reason to worry—little reason to think that my sister's disease would in the end have much to do with me. But I couldn't stop, wouldn't stop my search—and not only because I had promised my sister that I wouldn't. No; in fact, I didn't stop because this letter was so unsatisfying.

We know so much about cancer and disease relative to what we knew just a few decades ago that we often fail to comprehend how little we understand of the complete picture. Scientists have isolated two genes they believe to be linked to breast and ovarian cancers, but there most certainly are other genes and other causes working alone or in tandem. We base our disease history on the vague medical diagnoses that were available when our forebearers died and take comfort that a disease does not run in our family—or at least not that we know of. And except in the rare case of acute workplace toxicity, doctors almost never ask or comment on environmental factors that may be associated with our health histories—a fact that leaves a glaring, gaping hole in my history.

My own choices were stark, and the medical literature was not all that helpful. Though I had given up on being able to have a second child, I still needed to decide whether to have my ovaries removed. Although in the grand statistical scheme of things my sister's disease had doubled my chance of eventually developing ovarian cancer, the risk was still small—between 2 and 6 percent—and the fact that I didn't have the well-known genetic markers made it unclear what those figures actually meant for me. The physicians were split. Some doctors recommended immediate removal of my ovaries. Too scary a disease to chance it, too hard to detect, went their reasoning. Others didn't think the data, with only one member of my immediate family exhibiting the illness, was enough to justify the operation.

I knew that I had been exposed to a mix of dangerous chemicals in my hometown—at least one of which had been banned as a probable human carcinogen. But this exposure was both hard to quantify and hard to understand. There are no scientific studies to gauge the overlapping effects of the chemicals I was exposed to, and there never will be. Chemicals, to the extent that they are tested at all for toxicity, are tested one at a time. There are no scientific tests for the chemical cocktails that exist in places like Waukegan.

Despite the persistent uncertainty, however, I had to make a choice. The doctors could and did disagree, politicians could and did argue over who was responsible for the pollution and the cleanup, scientists could and did dispute the exact amount of PCBs that were dangerous to human health. But for me, this was not an academic or a theoretical question. I had a decision to make and risks to weigh.

CHAPTER SEVEN

Miasma

THERE IS A WORD FOR
the particular kind of uncertainty I faced when confronted
with my own medical choices and with my sister's illness
and its possible roots in our heavily polluted town. *Miasma,*
a thick fog or haze. The word comes from the Greek and
loosely translated means "polluted." Today, economists and
stock analysts often use it to indicate that the information
surrounding a company has become polluted or untrustwor-
thy in a way that makes it hard to ascertain the company's
exact value or competitive position. Many observers, for
example, thought that a kind of information miasma had
formed around the Internet boom in the late 1990s, which
caused investors to rush into buying high-tech stocks, an
action they later came to regret.

The roots of the word, however, are more directly
related to disease. Back in the mid-1800s when coal-fired
furnaces heated homes and factories, before germs, viruses,
and DNA were fully understood, people used to believe that
diseases sprang forth from the thick haze of the city—a
miasma. *Malaria,* for example, means literally "bad air" (*mal*

for bad, *aria* for air). The very way in which disease was understood tied it to a particular place.[1]

Consider, for example, perhaps one of the most feared diseases of the mid-1800s, cholera. It was John Snow who invented the modern science of epidemiology, the study of the factors that affect health, when he famously tracked an outbreak of cholera to a water pump. Snow carefully mapped the occurrence of cholera cases in a London neighborhood, marking each house in which a death had occurred with a black bar and noting its location in relation to the town's water wells. Working backward from the charted deaths, he correctly surmised that water from a certain well was causing the disease. Removing the handle to the pump was sufficient to stop the spread of the disease. The cause and the cure were both localized.

Today, however, we live in a vastly more complex world. Disease moves swiftly through populations, even from one continent to another, with the rapid and frequent movement of goods and people across borders. Swine flu, avian flu, mad cow disease, and AIDS are all examples of the swift spread of disease across continents and in time. Cancers, with lead times of twenty, thirty, or forty years from cause to malignancy, can be even harder to trace. The cause may be the radiant glow of the sun on a child in Australia, but the disease itself, a malignant melanoma of the skin, will not bloom until many years later, and by then it will show itself in the boy turned banker who is now a middle-aged worker in an office building on Wall Street. As a result, the relationship between disease and place is often murky or lost entirely. Instead, in our global, borderless world, disease, especially if it is one that flowers decades after its seeds are planted, may seem to exist on its own—isolated and divorced from any particular place and often from any apparently distinct cause.

Science itself has helped drive a wedge between place and disease. Today we understand disease at its most basic level—the virus, the bacteria, the exact cellular changes that mark this cancer or that one. Our vast knowledge about the way that illness infiltrates the body has led us to isolate disease in the lab, on the swab, the slide, the tissue sample, or cached only in particular cells. From this perspective, disease—if it is rooted in any place at all—is at home only in the body, and then only in one individual body.[2]

And when there is actually more connection between place and disease than meets the eye, a question inevitably arises: why, with the massive amounts of pollution in Waukegan, didn't a lot of people get visibly and noticeably sick? This was the question I sought to answer as a young reporter trying to understand what had happened to my town.

When I first started writing about Waukegan and the lakefront pollution after my sister died in 1995, I thought the effects of the chemicals would show themselves powerfully within the community. I expected that if I looked carefully enough I would find a smoking gun, a perfect epidemiological study such as the one Snow had done with his cholera. If I mapped the cases of cancer and then drew links to the way the wind blew from the lake, say, it would reveal a small epidemic. Or if I could find the right plant manager, he would lead me to a series of cases that were related in one form or another to the fluid that dripped onto the floor in the factories. Or maybe a really smart graduate student had happened on just the right piece of evidence and had written a breathtaking paper. Perhaps my old family physician in

Waukegan would recall a pattern of disease that would lead me to the certainty I was looking for.

Naively and tentatively I began my search by knocking on the door of a small trailer, an outpost of the town's health department. The kind woman at the door only shook her head when asked about the effects of fish in the water. She had fliers in pink and white promoting early screening for breast and cervical cancer. They were in Spanish and English. She thought that perhaps there were more cervical cancers than usual, but no, she didn't think the reason lay either in the fish or the water.

Downtown at the library where I studied as a girl, I asked the librarian, who told me a story about her father-in-law who had developed asbestosis after working in the Johns-Manville plant for just one year. She led me downstairs to a small, dark room. We pushed past some boxes and in disarray lay the paper trail the U.S. EPA had created when they documented the hazardous contents of each polluted site. Every chemical and its possible effects were recorded, but there were no records on public-health problems in the town.

I went to the Lake County Health Department too. They told me they had once tried to start a study on low-birthweight babies, but were denied the grant that would have funded it. I called on the historical society where the librarian chided me: "They didn't exactly put things like that in the paper, you know. They just called it cancer and didn't worry about what had caused it."

I asked her if she remembered the Never Rest Farm, where my family had bought vegetables. She did recall a farm on Lewis Avenue near our house, and she called a friend who still lived nearby to confirm its location using their combined memories. With old maps and phone books, we tried to site the farm exactly. We concluded that it was south of the bowling alley and before you got to the high-tension power lines that come from the coal-fired power plant on the lake. That would put it near the current Wendy's fast-food restaurant and adjacent to the Yeoman Creek Superfund site—pretty much exactly where I remembered it.

Later, as we pored over old newspapers, the librarian told me that quite a few years ago, when the sites were still stinking and the lawsuits being filed, lawyers representing the companies on the lake had visited the historical society and taken away many documents and artifacts. Then, with a quiet display of ladylike defiance, she showed me a piece she hadn't let the lawyers take away. Wrapped in a plastic bag was a small invitation to a gala on the lakefront celebrating a production milestone. It was made entirely out of asbestos fiber, so it looked something like a floor tile with fancy printing, its toxic dust smudging the bag. "I better put it away now," she said after I looked at it for a couple of minutes.

Like everyone in town, this woman knew someone who had been ill. A man who had worked one summer in a plant on the lakefront seemed never to be the same, children who developed rashes, the kid next door who didn't seem to be able to learn. The stories were always like that: intriguing, but difficult to pin down. There was always someone somewhere with something. Like the miasmas of yesteryear, disease was, well, in the air.

My investigation was complicated by the fact that, as the factories closed, many former plant workers of my father's generation and my schoolmates scattered. With no potential for work, they moved elsewhere, taking their health histories and any links to the town's pollution with them.

Epidemiology is a notoriously weak science. It typically takes large numbers of affected people to provide robust evidence for even small correlations of cause and effect, and the shifting population in my hometown made such connections impossible. That town officials have always downplayed pollution in the region and the associated health threats also meant that there was no one to agitate for further study of the area. Indeed, town officials have steadfastly refused to believe that the chemicals might have ever hurt anyone. Asked recently if anyone had come back and suggested they had gotten sick from the pollution in Waukegan, the mayor said, "No, not anyone, not ever. How long do we have to wait?"[3]

I didn't tell him my story, or my sister's. But I might have told him he didn't have to wait any longer. I might have said, today, right now, right here. You are looking at one person made sick by what happened here. But I knew that my story would be unlikely to sway him. To a large extent, we choose what we want to believe.

We also choose to create our own ignorance and then cling to it, in the same way we choose to create knowledge and cherish it. We decide which links to explore and which ones to bury. Writing about her own cancer in *Living Downstream*, the biologist Sandra Steingraber went searching for links between her disease and the broad agricultural fields covered with pesticides and herbicides in southern Illinois where she grew up. She found that while the state's cancer registry was established, funded, and thriving, its stillborn twin, the hazardous substance registry, was not:

> The environment, it seems, keeps falling off the cancer screen. The circumstances surrounding the birth of the Illinois State Cancer Registry is a case in point.

The registry came into being when the Illinois Health and Hazardous Substances Registry Act was signed by the governor in September 1984. As implied by its name, this state law was intended to "monitor the health effects among the citizens of Illinois related to exposures to hazardous substances in the work place and in the environment." Accordingly, the registry system was to collect information not only on the incidence of cancer among the Illinois populace but also on their "exposure to hazardous substances, including hazardous nuclear material," thus prompting public health studies that would relate "measurable health outcomes to environmental data to help identify contributing factors in the occurrence of disease."

The cancer registry was funded. The hazardous substances registry was not.[4]

Without the hazardous substances registry, half the story was missing. If the records had been kept, if the Waukegan Historical Society files had not been searched and removed, if people had stayed in place, what might we know about the links between the environment and health? More, certainly, than we do now.

The Illinois State Cancer Registry, for example, suggests that there is slightly more non-Hodgkin's lymphoma in the county surrounding my hometown than there is in other Illinois counties. Non-Hodgkin's lymphoma is a cancer that a federal toxics agency suggests may be associated with PCB exposure. But without a detailed study of where the disease occurred and to whom, it would be hard to make a link between the exposures and the cancers.

Determining what we know and what we cannot know,

the precise nature and causes of our uncertainty, is a fundamental aspect of any inquiry. The poet Rainer Maria Rilke once suggested to a young author that, in the absence of answers, he had only one choice: to learn to love the questions themselves as if they were locked rooms or books written in a foreign language. That was the situation I found myself in.

Having no ready answers, I had no choice but to love the questions. Lacking a grand, bulletproof epidemiological study of Waukegan's population, I had this left to consider: there are studies of workers exposed in factories, there are studies of those who eat Great Lakes fish, there are accidental exposures such as those from contaminated rice oil in Japan, and there are animal studies. From these we must draw conclusions that, of necessity, are more guarded and less direct than we might have hoped, but no less valid reasons for concern.

Decades of research sponsored by the federal Agency for Toxic Substances and Disease Registry (ATSDR), charged by Congress to study the effects of toxic chemicals in the Great Lakes, found the following effects related to PCBs:

1. Reproductive function may be disrupted by exposure to PCBs, including shortened menstrual cycles and decreased fertility.
2. Neurobehavioral, learning, attention, and development deficits occur in newborns, and these deficits persist as the children reach school age. The most highly exposed children were three times more likely to have low verbal IQ scores and were twice as likely to lag behind in reading comprehension.

3. Other systemic effects (e.g., self-reported liver disease and diabetes, and effects on the thyroid and immune systems) are associated with elevated serum levels of PCBs.

4. Increased cancer risk (e.g., non-Hodgkin's lymphoma) is associated with PCB exposure.[5]

After my visit to the Waukegan Historical Society, I drove behind the Wendy's where I remember the farm being. At the Superfund site behind the former farm, workers were stretching a black, impenetrable piece of plastic over the ground as the remediation reached completion stage. The hope is that the chemicals will forever remain sealed under the tarplike material. Their effects on my town were similarly buried when the factory workers moved away, the studies went unfunded, the files were removed, and the data was left unassembled.

We will never have a large-scale epidemiological study of the effects of the chemicals on Waukegan. That much is certain, and there are those who will dismiss the case I am making here as lacking statistical significance. That would be a mistake.

Long before there were statistics or scientific studies, there were stories—stories that warned of the link between environmental factors and their potential health effects. Shepherds, for example, knew long before scientists proved it that some forms of clover made their sheep infertile, and so they relentlessly herded the animals from the pastures where it grew. As nations industrialized, natural elements like lead, coal, and petroleum, previously hidden underground, became common workplace irritants and cause for community concern; new links between place and disease were forged, and cautionary tales emerged. The phrase "mad as a hatter"—famously used by Lewis Carroll in *Alice in Wonderland*—dates to the nineteenth century, when it was coined to describe hat-factory workers poisoned by the mercury used in the hat production process. It is through the telling and retelling of stories that the lessons of individual illnesses have become fused into a common wisdom—a kind of health policy for the ages.

In our borderless world, the relationship between disease and place is no longer fixed. And our cultural connections between place and health have been unnaturally severed. As a result, we lack the stories of earlier years that warned us of hazardous plants and materials and that told of their disease-causing properties. It is only through telling scientifically based, carefully crafted stories that place and disease can be reunited. In this context, even individual stories matter.

Stories like my sister's, when studied closely, can sometimes speak volumes. The legendary cancer researcher Judah Folkman, who until his death headed the vascular-biology program at Children's Hospital in Boston, told the *Wall Street Journal* in 2006 that for many years he followed four patients with rare tumors who had taken an experimental drug. "There will be people who will dismiss the data, saying it is only four patients, but if you ask good questions you can learn a lot from a single patient," said Folkman. "The single patient can make you think differently."[6]

CHAPTER EIGHT

Hitchhiking Hormones

❧

CANCER TAKES MORE
than two hundred different forms, but all share the charac-
teristic of abnormal, unwanted, and unchecked growth of
cells. The now-common disease has been in evidence since
ancient times. The Greek medical writer Galen, for example, incorrectly attributed cancer to bad humors in the body,
but also perceptively noted that "cancerous tumors develop
with greatest frequency in the breast of women."[1]

In fact, until men started smoking and developing lung
cancer in noticeably large numbers in the twentieth century,
cancer was generally viewed as a woman's disease, and it
most often took the form of breast cancer.[2] "Throughout
much of human history," writes historian James Olson in
Bathsheba's Breast, "breast cancer was cancer."[3]

Historically, breast cancer was most often observed in
nuns, who were about five times more likely than other
women to die of the disease.[4] As far back as the 1700s, the
Italian physician Bernardino Ramazzini, a professor of
medicine at the University of Padua, noted the prevalence
of breast cancer among nuns, especially in contrast to the

relative rarity of the condition among women who had borne and suckled many children.[5]

The fact that Ramazzini and others observed the disease in nuns probably added to an incorrect notion that sexual repression, abstinence, or both contributed to the disease. It was a theory that lasted well into the twentieth century, when the poet W. H. Auden wrote about the churchgoing, straightlaced Miss Gee, who suffered from ovarian cancer.

Cancer's a funny thing.

Nobody knows what the cause is,
Though some pretend they do;
It's like some hidden assassin
Waiting to strike at you.

Childless women get it.
And men when they retire;
It's as if there had to be some outlet
For their foiled creative fire.[6]

Auden was wrong to attribute Miss Gee's ovarian cancer to lack of sexual fire, but he was correct in pointing out the correlation between the disease and a life without children. Modern researchers have found that women without children or women who bear children late in life are at higher risk for both ovarian and breast cancers. My only child was born when I was thirty-five, late enough for my pregnancy with him to be another risk factor for me to consider.

I learned a lot from my sister in our unscientific chats about sex, but that knowledge was not much help in my quest to understand her cancer, my own susceptibility, and the possibility that the chemicals in the lake were wreaking havoc with our health. So I found a textbook that I used in college and began studying ovaries.

"Ovaries are approximately three centimeters long by one and one-half centimeters wide by one centimeter thick," writes Ethel Sloan in *The Biology of Women.*[7] My edition of the book was a bland khaki copy that pictured a woman with an afro on the cover. The book was a feminist favorite during the 1980s, when groups of women studied it together to get in touch with our bodies. Today's version is graced by half a dozen goddesses in diaphanous dresses.

Whichever edition you consult will tell you that the ovary is about the size of an almond and that it produces the female hormone estrogen. During the monthly menstrual cycle, each ovary forces an egg through a wall of tissue and afterward repairs that rupture in a process called ovulation. "The ovary is no beauty," writes Natalie Angier in *Woman: An Intimate Geography.* "It is scarred and pitted, for each cycle of ovulation leaves behind a blemish where an egg follicle has been emptied of its contents. The older the woman, the more scarred her ovaries will be."[8] It is this continual bursting and repairing—part and parcel of the ovarian life cycle—that makes the ovary vulnerable to cancer.

Scientists have long theorized that as cells multiply each month to repair the breach in the ovarian wall, more opportunities are created for mistakes in the DNA copying process, which in turn increase the chances of a malignant mutation. More ovulations, in other words, mean more chances for mistakes.[9]

Risk factors for the disease therefore include never giving your ovaries a break by being pregnant or having a child. The other risk factor is having a close female relative with the disease. That would be my sister, of course, and that would bring the story back home.

Prior to my sister's illness, we had only one close relative with a related disease: my maternal grandmother's sister, our Great Aunt Alice, from whom I got my middle name. Aunt Alice graduated from a local college and worked as a secretary. I have pictures of her in a mink coat, smoking a cigarette. I think I would have liked her, but she died before I was born. But my sister recalled being taken into a dark, dusty room where Aunt Alice lay dying and whispering to the corpselike woman. It was an image she carried with her throughout her illness.

"I bet she had this," my sister would say.

We didn't check at the time, and today I am at a loss to explain our disinterest. Maybe we knew it didn't matter for my sister. Sue already had ovarian cancer, what difference would it make what Aunt Alice had? As a result of my uncharacteristic laziness and fear, I didn't try to find Aunt Alice's death certificate until I enrolled in the high-risk cancer clinic at a Boston hospital.

When the clinic asked me to bring in a complete family medical history on my second visit, my reporting skills kicked in. I had a task and deadline. I called the funeral director in Waukegan. After briefly remembering my mother and others in the family in a polite and solemn conversation, he located my aunt's death certificate and sent me a copy.

So here is what I had when I went to my second appointment at the clinic: my sister's slides, her pathology report and about a hundred pages of her records, my own records, and my aunt's newly copied death certificate.

The first woman I saw this time was a breast cancer specialist. She was wearing a red suit and sported a stylishly short haircut. I handed her Aunt Alice's death certificate with the diagnosis that meant nothing to me: "Cancer of the Peritoneal Cavity." My Aunt Alice died when she was forty-four years old. "She definitely had it," said the red-coated doctor and handed it back to me in a heartbeat.

She explained. The peritoneum is the lining that holds the internal organs. Since the ovaries brush up against the peritoneal lining and their cells are similar in nature, a diagnosis of peritoneal cancer is considered the equivalent of ovarian cancer—especially given that my aunt died in the early 1950s, before many of today's medical imaging techniques might have led to a more exact diagnosis. Now I had two relatives with the disease and a screeching headache. I stopped for a donut and headed to my next appointment to see an ovarian cancer specialist.

Doctors at this hospital and elsewhere have long speculated that there were significant environmental factors associated with ovarian cancer. The vagina provides a runway to the ovaries not simply for sperm but for many other substances as well. Significantly, women who have their tubes tied experience a lower rate of ovarian cancer than those who do not. Some have theorized that this may be because the pathway to the ovaries has been blocked, keeping outside agents at bay.[10]

For example, some researchers have found a link between talcum powder and ovarian cancer—though several other studies have produced conflicting results.[11] However, the discrepancy is a subtle one. Some early forms of talcum may have contained asbestos and thus given researchers their positive findings. Indeed, at least one retrospective study found a much higher disease rate among those women who used talc prior to 1960 than those who used it after—giving at least some credence to the idea that the use of asbestos-laden talc increases a woman's risk of ovarian cancer.

My sister speculated that asbestos had contributed to

her illness. A group of naturally occurring fibrous materials that are fire-resistant, asbestos has been thought to cause adverse health effects since the first century. Yet, as writer Paul Brodeur tells us in his book on asbestos, *Outrageous Misconduct*, its role in causing the disease asbestosis, a noncancerous condition in which the lungs scar so badly that they won't expand and contract properly, was not well established in the medical literature until the 1970s.

In the years before my sister died, when I was an editor at the *Harvard Business Review*, I worked on a piece written by Bill Sells, the man who had run the Johns-Manville plant in Waukegan in the early 1970s—a time when deaths from asbestosis and other asbestos-related diseases were beginning to occur in the workforce at an alarming rate. After noting that his job included the unenviable task of visiting his sick and dying employees at the local hospital, he offered this description of his first visit to the factory: "The plant lay at the back of a sprawling complex built in the 1920s. Its view of Lake Michigan was obscured by a landfill several stories high. A road wound through this mountain of asbestos-laden scrap, and as I drove through it for the first time I stopped to watch a bulldozer crush a 36-inch sewer pipe. A cloud of dust swirled around my car." Inside the plant, he said, he found "asbestos-laden dust coating almost every visible surface."[12]

An EPA official charged with overseeing the cleanup of the Johns-Manville plant, Brad Bradley, has a similar recollection. Standing at the edge of the 350-acre Superfund site that overlooks Lake Michigan, Bradley recalled his first visit there in 1982. He remembers asking an asbestos expert where he thought they would find the fibers. "I think they are everywhere," said the expert. Indeed, virtually anywhere on the site that Bradley scuffed the ground with his boot, he found the telltale fibers.

People are more likely to connect the fiber with asbestosis than with ovarian cancer. However, a thirty-year study of nearly two thousand women who worked with asbestos while manufacturing gas masks during World War II showed these women to be seven times more likely to die from ovarian cancer than a control group.[13] My sister's medical history seems to tell a different story, though, and the link between asbestos and ovarian cancer in general does not appear to be a strong one. The ovarian cancer specialist I saw at the clinic was quick to point out that my sister's record indicated that her cancer was preceded by endometriosis.

The phrase "painful periods" does not begin to describe the torture that my mother and sister endured during menstruation. White and sweating, doubled over with pain, they retreated to the bed or the couch until the pain and the bleeding passed. When I recounted my mother's experience, the ovarian cancer specialist suggests that my mother also likely suffered from endometriosis.

Endometriosis is a once rare disease that is now common. When the disease was first named and discovered in 1921 by a New York physician, there were only twenty reports of the illness in the medical literature.[14] Today, the National Institutes of Health estimates that roughly 5.5 million women suffer from the disease in the United States, and as many as 89 million women may have it worldwide. An exact number is hard to come by, since the disease can only properly be diagnosed during surgery. Still, about one-third of women of childbearing age suffer some symptoms—including pelvic pain and infertility—and in the United States at least, the average age of onset has been declining.[15]

The increasing occurrence of endometriosis is in part due to improved diagnostic techniques and the fact that doctors are more willing to see menstrual pain as a real health issue. However, the growth in the number of diagnoses also points to a true increase in the prevalence of the problem.

Endometriosis is a complex condition, and no one is certain what causes it. Some scientists believe it is an immune system disorder. Others believe that women with endometriosis lack the ability to shed cells that have migrated and are growing where they should not be. Other scientists have focused on a genetic component of the disease, since it can run in families. A woman with a sister or mother with endometriosis, for example, is three to seven times more likely to get the disease.[16]

The mechanisms of endometriosis are not that different from those that create cancer: they involve cell proliferation, the migration of cells, and a change in their cellular nature. Endometriosis grows unchecked and invades surrounding tissues, and the body's immune system fails to rid itself of the misplaced lesions. In the same way, the body fails to rid itself of cancerous lesions.

It is often but not always the case that the kind of cancer my sister suffered from, ovarian clear-cell adenocarcinoma, is preceded by endometriosis, and many believe that there is a relationship between the two diseases. Some scientists believe that endometriosis—in certain cases—is a kind of precancerous condition, and others believe that the two diseases spring forth in unison. Other experts theorize that the endometrial cells themselves drive the proliferation of cancer once it has started by producing their own estrogen. Each lesion is capable of increasing the local production of estrogen, so that once the disease takes hold it is capable of feeding itself.

In my sister's case, cancerous growths arose within her endometrial lesions. Whatever the exact mechanism of disease development, women with the type of ovarian cancer that my sister suffered from have higher rates of endometriosis than the general female population. In one study, about 70 percent of the women with clear-cell ovarian cancer also had endometriosis.[17]

Scientists have long suspected that chemicals of the type found in Waukegan—dioxins, PCBs, and polycyclic aromatic hydrocarbons (PAHs)—play a role in human endometriosis. The evidence is most compelling in relation to the 210 known dioxins. Dioxins are chemicals with similar toxicologic effects that are never made intentionally, but rather are by-products of many industrial processes. A small subset of PCBs have dioxin-like effects.[18] Both PCBs and dioxins are endocrine disruptors, and dioxin-like chemicals—including PCBs—have consistently been linked to the development of endometriosis in tests performed on laboratory animals.

Female monkeys have reproductive organs and menstrual cycles similar to women, and so they make for excellent test subjects. In a study conducted by scientists at Vanderbilt University and Dartmouth College, monkeys injected with a single dose of dioxin later showed high rates of endometriosis—indeed, several had such severe cases of the disorder that they died from it. Interestingly, the monkeys showed blood levels of dioxins and PCBs equal to those that a woman might carry from everyday exposures to chemicals in food and the air.[19]

Two recent studies in humans confirm a link between PCBs and endometriosis. One study of eighty women conducted in Rome found that women diagnosed with endometriosis had 1.6 times higher blood levels of PCBs than women without the disease. The other study found that levels of four particular types of PCBs were 3.77 times higher in women with endometriosis than in a control group of women who did not have the disease.[20]

These results are consistent with another finding—that women who live close to contaminated Great Lakes areas show a greater rate of hospitalization for endometriosis. A study done by Health Canada, for example, shows that women who live near Thunder Bay on Lake Superior—a place that has battled its own dioxin problem—are four times as likely to be hospitalized for endometriosis as those elsewhere in the province.[21]

Mary Lou Ballweg is founder and president of the Wisconsin-based Endometriosis Association. Both a victim of the disease and an ardent advocate in the fight against it, she believes from the evidence she has examined that the link between Great Lakes pollution and endometriosis is a strong one.

While we can never know exactly what levels of what chemicals existed in my sister's bloodstream or mine years ago, we can approximate them by looking at general statistics for people who lived in the Great Lakes area. A 2005 report by the Centers for Disease Control and Prevention, the federal agency that tracks the amounts of various pollutants in the bloodstream of Americans, found that those who ate Great Lakes fish had concentrations of PCBs and dioxins that were several times the concentrations in the general population.[22]

Why do PCBs have such an effect on reproductive organs? In an unusual twist of fate, PCB molecules are shaped in such a way that they bind to the estrogen receptors in the cells of ovarian tissue. Dioxins and the structurally related polycyclic aromatic hydrocarbons also bind to receptors—known informally as dioxin receptors—in the cells that make up ovarian tissue. PCBs, dioxins, and PAHs are thus able to accumulate in ovarian structures and fluids, disrupting ovary development and ovulation. Working alone or in tandem, these synthetic estrogens and anti-estrogens are believed to promote infertility; they have also been shown to promote ovarian tumors in animals. Because they disrupt the natural production of estrogen, they may also play a role in endometriosis.

Because these chemicals are able to disturb the endocrine system and the production of hormones in the body, they are known as endocrine disruptors. Endocrine disruptors are external agents that interfere with the functioning of natural hormones in the body.

Theo Colborn, who began her scientific career studying endocrine-disrupting chemicals in the Great Lakes, put it this way in a book she coauthored, *Our Stolen Future*: "Hormonally active synthetic chemicals are thugs on the biological information highway that sabotage vital communication. They mug the messengers or impersonate them. They jam signals. They scramble messages. They sow disinformation. They wreak all manor of havoc."[23]

Given the extent of the animal data and what is known about the role of dioxin receptors, coupled with the fact that my sister would have been exposed to these chemicals on a variety of occasions, it is biologically plausible, if not definitive, that dioxin, PCBs, and PAHs could interact with human ovarian cells and ovarian function in such a manner as to induce or promote the development of endometriosis and ovarian cancer.

And while the studies I found weren't exactly the smoking gun I had been looking for, they were impressive enough that I wanted to step up my own screening for ovarian cancer. Even if I didn't know the exact mechanism by which the chemicals in Lake Michigan may have made my sister sick, I had a pretty good hunch. I also had a strong suspicion that those very same chemicals had contributed to my infertility. What other effects, I wondered, might they eventually have on my body?

CHAPTER NINE

Me Too

꩜

Screening seems like such an innocent, costless sort of thing—unless you have ever had to do it. Screening implies just checking in on things every once in awhile, the way you might peek in on a sleeping child. But unlike the warmth that fills you when you look at your sleeping baby, a screening test provides brief comfort and much anxiety—even a clean test, after all, serves only to confirm that you are at risk.

"These check-ups represent the background of illness shading back into the foreground," writes Arthur Frank, a Canadian sociologist and cancer survivor. "Even for those whose visa is stamped expeditiously, the reality of lacking permanent citizenship is reaffirmed."[1]

You lose weeks in this process, too. First, the weeks before the appointment, scheduling and rescheduling it, to make sure you have time for the emotional overload it will create. Assiduously avoiding birthdays, anniversaries, school plays, and teacher conferences, you settle on a date. The test itself might be fast, or you might wait for hours as I once did, when each of the three women before me was diagnosed with breast cancer—a day that left the staff weeping in a darkened hallway.[2]

Then you lose days after the test, waiting for the phone to ring, the doctor to call, the letter to come. You spend your days remembering over and over the faces of the technicians and the receptionists, searching your mind to conjure up a reassuring fact, phrase, or expression.

"Whether she expresses it overtly or somehow manages the outward appearance of composure, nothing less than a physician's reassurance that all is well can put a halt to the frightening wanderings of her imagination," writes the physician Sherwin Nuland of the patient undergoing screening. "She has read too much, and perhaps experienced too much, to approach this part of the physical examination with anything resembling a serene mind. At the very least, she will fear surgery, disfigurement, and the discomforts of therapy. Her anxieties may reach much further, to terrifying fantasies that involve the loss of self-esteem, love and life itself."[3]

And that, dear doctor, is a best-case scenario. Screening for me involves a kind of blank terror. No thoughts, just plain old white-knuckled panic.

In March 2003, some eleven years after my sister was first diagnosed with ovarian cancer and just before I was about to make another pilgrimage home to Illinois to do more research, I bravely scheduled another screening for ovarian cancer. During the ultrasound procedure, the doctor slipped a small tube into my vagina, and my uterus and ovaries appeared on the screen. I liked this particular doctor because he was fast and, unlike most doctors, he talked while he worked. Usually he would reassure me, saying that looks fine, all normal there, as he moved the wand with one hand and snapped pictures with another. Once he even congratulated me on my textbook ovaries.

Let me tell you what every high-risk cancer patient knows. If you screen for it, you will find it, whatever it is, even if it is nothing at all, which it usually is. Until that day when it is something so big and so dramatic that your favorite radiologist says part in prayer, part in astonishment: "Jesus Christ, what is that?"

The moment I heard his words, I knew what it was. It was the disease I had been thinking about, studying, and writing about since I promised my sister I would write about her cancer.

I left the radiologist's office shaken and fearful. Just moments out of the parking lot, my cell phone rang. It was my personal physician calling from the hospital. She asked me if the radiologist told me how big the cyst was. "Yes," I said, "nine centimeters long." Almost four inches.

"Are you sure he didn't say nine millimeters?" she asked sternly.

Yes, I said, I was sure. Still, she could not believe the report she was reading.

"Well at least we don't have to kid ourselves that we found it early," I said in an attempt at humor. She didn't laugh. Instead she ordered more tests for the next day.

One of those tests confirmed the size of the cyst, but was unable to locate its origins—everyone's best guess was that it was coming from the rear of my peritoneum, the sack that holds my abdominal organs. Aunt Alice's weird, archaic diagnosis rang in my head; I was sure that I had the disease that killed both my aunt and my sister. My doctors were less certain.

So they asked me to sign a release form allowing the

surgeon to remove my colon, my spleen, my pancreas, and assorted lymph nodes. An administrator reviewing my admission asked pointedly: "Don't they know what they are going to do?" I tried to explain, but stopped. They had no idea what they would find when they opened my abdomen.

The day before my surgery, I ran a thousand small errands—screen repairs, dry cleaning, and, of course, I vacuumed the minivan, which is always, always dirty. Cleaning is the defensive action of all moms in trouble. It works.

In a three-hour-long surgery, the doctors discovered a four-inch-long mucus-filled cyst attached to the end of my pancreas. Officially, it is called a mucinous cystadenocarcinoma. It is, rather unpoetically, a large, grapefruit-sized sac filled with snot.

It was two weeks before the tests confirmed my worst fear. The four-inch cyst held a one-and-one-half-centimeter cancerous spot. The cancer, however, had not spread. It was confined within my cyst. The doctor removed 70 percent of my pancreas, my spleen, and a lymph node for good measure. There was no cancer in any of these organs or tissues. My sister's diagnosis came on April 3, 1992; she was forty-one. My diagnosis came eleven years and one day later, on April 4, 2003; I was forty-three.

"This just cannot be a coincidence," said one of my many doctors after learning of my pancreatic cancer. He has been my doctor since I joined the high-risk clinic after my sister's cancer was diagnosed. His words echoed my worst fears and the best instincts of the Harvard-trained genealogist down the hall, who simply shook her head and said with words trailing off into a whisper, "Two sisters with rare cancers in their forties . . ."

Yet there is no known familial syndrome that can explain

our diseases, and repeated and exhaustive genetic testing for known mutations, including for the now well-known BRCA breast cancer gene, has revealed no relevant genetic links that would help explain either my own or my sister's cancer. My doctors, noting that they cannot adequately explain the origins of either cancer, offered this in a formal letter that came several weeks later: "Cancer can cluster in a family for several reasons including shared environmental exposures, similar lifestyles and random bad luck."[4]

My sister and I shared a similar lifestyle that included a love for vegetables, yoga, and our children. Neither of us drank or smoked. Mostly we shared one enormous set of toxic environmental exposures in Waukegan, Illinois.

"Illness is not presented to the ill as a moral problem," writes Arthur Frank, who has written beautifully about his own illness. "People are not asked, after the shock of diagnosis has dulled sufficiently, what do you wish to become in this experience? What story do you wish to tell of yourself? How will you shape your illness, and yourself, in the stories you tell of it?"[5]

And yet that was the dilemma I faced. Most people are not in the midst of writing a book about the origins of their sister's cancer when their own cancer is discovered. I was. And even if it seems too much like a TV movie to be true, it was, well, true.

I had gone from a patient at high risk to a card-carrying, bracelet-wearing, bona fide cancer patient. My story was my sister's once over. My kind of cancer, pancreatic, is more deadly and at least as stealthy as ovarian. About 2 percent of all new cancer diagnoses each year are pancreatic—about twenty-eight thousand cases. Ninety-seven percent of people diagnosed with the disease die within five years; half of them die within the first six months.[6] I was lucky, however, in that I developed a rare kind of pancreatic cancer that gives me an uncertain, but much more hopeful, prognosis. That kind, mucinous cystadenocarcinoma, represents just 5.7 percent of all pancreatic cancers, and few doctors see even a handful of patients of this type.[7] In fact, one senior doctor at a leading hospital ventured that there have been only fifty or so cases in his entire hospital ever.

Noninvasive pancreatic cancers of this type are almost always cured by surgery alone. However, in my case, the cancerous cells had begun to grow into the lining of my cyst. As such, my case was borderline, deemed "microinvasive" despite the fact that my lymph nodes and the areas of my pancreas that bordered the tumor were free of disease. Had the disease spread to the lymph nodes or the tissue around the tumor, or to the pancreas itself, the disease would likely recur and would possibly morph into the much more deadly form of pancreatic cancer—ductal adenocarcinoma.

My doctors were not shy about telling me that if my cancer were to reoccur in my pancreas and change into that more serious kind of cancer, the results would be lethal. There are only a handful of cases where this reoccurrence has taken place.[8] Ominously, one case study originated in the prestigious hospital where I received treatment. The doctors who handled the case are among the best known in the nation and are colleagues of my doctors. This story spooked everyone—especially me.

"Incurable," said my oncologist, uttering a word all but banned in a cancer hospital. "If that happens, if your cancer returns in its most deadly form, it will be incurable."

Oncologists can be at times charming, at times intimidating, even ruthless. My doctor was certain that I should do chemotherapy in the aftermath of my operation. Perhaps because I had witnessed my sister's treatments, I was hesitant, scared, and indecisive.

He recommended that I undergo a twenty-four-week course of chemotherapy with a drug named 5-FU. Other high-ranking physicians at the same cancer hospital did not agree. One doctor called chemotherapy in my case "superstitious" and of unknown benefit. This doctor is beyond famous; his name shows up regularly in the pages of the *New York Times*, a fact that only further threw me into a tizzy. Other doctors were more radical and recommended that I have a large portion of my abdomen irradiated—a process that would likely leave me with kidney damage. Everyone but a few fringe physicians seemed to think this was quite literally overkill.

The catch phrase in hospitals today is *evidence-based medicine*, or EBM. In practicing evidence-based medicine, doctors attempt to uniformly apply what they have learned from science when prescribing treatment to individual patients who share the same or a similar disease. This works well when there are large numbers of people who have been diagnosed with a well-studied disease, say, breast or lung cancer. It works less well when there is scant evidence and doctors have differing opinions about the small amount of evidence that exists.

In the end, it was my choice and my choice alone what to do. Searching for more opinions simply added up the tallies on my chemo scorecard, with no consensus emerging.

I hated the idea of chemotherapy and hated even more the idea of dying and leaving my son alone. Moreover, I simply hated the idea of choosing. A study in the *Journal of Clinical Epidemiology* in 1992 found that although 64 percent of the general public believes they want to make their own choices about cancer treatment, only 12 percent of newly diagnosed cancer patients actually want to.9

My situation has been dramatized on dozens of TV shows, argued over in courtrooms, and written about by the ill, the famous, and the erudite at least since the eighteenth century, when the English poet Alexander Pope, himself a sufferer from severe illness, penned his oft-quoted line: "Who shall decide, when doctors disagree?"

While I cannot settle a debate that has raged for centuries, I can say this with certainty. In today's patient-driven, cost-conscious, litigious medical world, when the evidence is nonexistent, it is the patient who decides. In my mind, the decision itself defied logic. You either needed chemo or you didn't. *Elective* is not a word that should be attached to chemotherapy, but in my case it was.

The odds that any of the cancerous cells had escaped from my tumor were small, maybe 1–2 percent, but real. When doctors do a biopsy they can only look carefully, microscopically, at a small section. From that section they must generalize. When pathologists studied a small section of my tumor, they found that the cancerous cells had invaded the outer lining of the tumor. The question was, did any escape? No one was certain. Could they have? Absolutely. Could there have been other undetected cancerous spots where the cells might have escaped? You bet. That's why the doctors suggested I undergo what they call adjuvant chemotherapy, just-in-case chemotherapy. The hitch was that no one knew whether chemotherapy would be effective in a case like mine.10

"The only certainty I have learned in a long career in

medicine is this," writes the physician Sherwin Nuland in *The Wisdom of the Body*. "A disease presents itself in a unique form in each person it attacks, and it pursues a unique course. A prognosis is a statement of probability, not of fact."[11]

I grilled my doctor about his recommendation again and again. Why didn't the other eminent doctors in his hospital, the chairman of his department even, feel it necessary? How could he be so adamant, so certain?

His answer was simple and to the point. The other doctors didn't have to look me in the eye. They wouldn't be the ones to tell me the deadly disease was back, if indeed it did come back. He couldn't stand it if the disease came back and it was, as he predicted, incurable. The others could take the scientific high ground, exhibit best-practices bravado, play the odds. The two of us, however, were not playing at all.

I decided to do it. Not to be heroic, since I could just as easily argue that what I was doing was unnecessary. Not because I love my son and my husband beyond belief, because no matter how much you love someone you simply cannot live forever for them no matter how hard you try. In the end, I chose to do it because I wanted to live.

In some strange coincidence, the administrators at the hospital picked the anniversary of my sister's death as the date to commence treatment. "Too weird," said my husband, urging me to find another date. I agreed and rescheduled. I settled on a fine summer day in June 2003 after my son had finished school for the year.

Since my cancer is not well studied, the doctors and I decided on a course of treatment that is the standard prescribed therapy for a much more common cancer, colon cancer. Even if the drug in question has not been tested for efficacy in my situation, it has been tested and used many times over on thousands of people. In other words, there is evidence that the drug is safe—as safe as taking any poison can be.

Throughout my treatment, I wanted the drug—called 5-FU—to mean, fuck you five times over. I imagined some drug researcher working hard to save a family member in the grips of this horrible disease. I imagined her whispering into the night fuck you, fuck you, fuck you, as she worked late in her lab—hexing the disease even as she conquered it. My story about the origins of the drug was way off. Truth, it turns out, is stranger than fiction or the drug-induced fantasies of chemotherapy patients.

The first chemotherapy drugs were distilled from the roots of the mayapple (*Podophyllum peltatum*), a common woodland plant in the northeastern United States and Canada. Although its tumor-suppressing properties were not well known until the 1860s, the extract made from the plant appears in the medical materials list of the first U.S. pharmacopoeia published in the 1820s—making it officially the first chemotherapy in America.[12]

Modern chemotherapy as we know it, though, has far more nefarious roots. It comes from the waging of modern war, more specifically, from the study and use of mustard gas in World War I and an explosion in World War II. Mustard gas was most famously used by the Germans in the Belgian city of Ypres in 1917 and thus is sometimes given the name Yperite. It gives rise to oozing blisters that secrete a mustard-yellow pus (hence its more common name). Soldiers who were exposed also oozed mucus from their eyes, and some eventually went blind—which is why in John

Singer Sargent's famous portrait *Gassed* the men are blind-
folded, stumbling in a line through the fallen bodies of their
compatriots.[13]

Early studies in the United States indicated that mustard gas had a powerful cell toxicity, but it wasn't until World
War II that the medicinal properties of the gas were discovered in earnest. The freighter *John Harvey*, carrying one
hundred tons of mustard gas, was bombed in 1943 in a
southern Italian harbor. One thousand people perished
immediately; 617 survived with severe burns and other
effects from the gas.[14]

When bodies were shipped back to the United States
for further study, earlier studies of the cell toxicity of mustard gas were confirmed, and researchers at Yale moved
quickly to use the substance to treat patients with lymphoma.[15] "Americans got better at saving lives partly because
they got better at taking them," writes historian Edmund
Russell in his book *War and Nature*. "The fundamental biological principles of poisoning soldiers, insects, rats, bacteria, and cancer are essentially the same."[16]

Which, of course, leads to an obvious problem: taking a
poison even if it is meant to be a cure can be dangerous. Infusion wards are not unlike beauty parlors in some respects.
The patients sit in long lines of reclining chairs. Each person has a private area with curtains, although the whole
ward is visible from the nurses' station since at any time a
reaction to a drug could prove fatal. Crash carts stand read-
ied against the wall. All told, my treatments could take
between four and six hours, depending on how crowded the
ward was on a given day.

The nurses who administer the drugs wear large blue
gloves and sometimes black rubberized aprons, since even

a drop of the drug on your skin might burn you. If an infusion goes awry—that is, the drug does not drain directly into the vein and instead pools just under the skin, as mine often did—it leaves small burn marks up and down your arm.

One day during my treatment course, I was sitting in the big blue chair I favored because it was close to the window. After nurses had opened my veins, I opened the *New York Times*. Flipping through the front section of the paper, I came across a story about the Bush administration's decision to sell lands infused with PCBs. Here is the abstract of what I read.

E.P.A. Relaxes Restrictions on Sale of Contaminated Land

September 3, 2003
By JENNIFER LEE (NYT); National Desk

Washington, D.C. – EPA relaxes restrictions on selling some land contaminated with PCBs for redevelopment; says restrictions are unnecessary barrier to economic redevelopment and may actually delay cleanup of contaminated properties; change does not affect most severely PCB-contaminated sites covered by Superfund law; environmental groups say shift is part of pattern at EPA that is making it easier to redevelop contaminated sites at expense of public health.[17]

As I read the article, my brain did a little dance of shivering disbelief. The cancer-causing properties of PCBs are well-known; recent scientific reviews have only confirmed the chemicals' toxicity. In fact, current scientific work suggests these chemicals have the potential to disrupt the body's hormones and weaken the immune system in such a way that could potentially promote a cancer's spread. The chemicals were banned in 1976, some twenty-seven years before the *New York Times* article was written, precisely because PCBs had been shown to create tumors in animals and Great Lakes fish. In the years since, as our knowledge of genetics, cellular mechanisms, and toxicity has improved, the evidence that these chemicals are dangerous has continued to mount.

So there I was, sitting in a room with about thirty other people valiantly trying to kill our cancer cells while the government was releasing lands contaminated with chemicals that were known to cause and promote cancer. Sometimes the personal and the political are so closely fused that they become inseparable. Anger coursed through my veins along with the chemo drugs. Suddenly a wave of nausea swept over me. I wondered if it was the news or the chemo. I couldn't stomach either.

As it turned out, I reached a point where I literally could not tolerate chemo. Each patient's reaction to chemotherapy seems to differ, just as it does to other substances, toxic or not. Some tolerate it well; others not at all. "I did just fine," says Mike Gall, a toxicologist at the Cancer Institute in New Jersey who was treated for non-Hodgkin's lymphoma. "But in the room right next to me is a person with the same disease, the same age, the same physique, and he's getting the stuffing kicked out of him. Why? My drug-metabolizing enzymes must be slightly different from his."[18]

For me, the first treatments went fine, but halfway into my course of treatment I developed a serious rash over half my body and was forced to stop. We were attending a Yom

Kippur service when my son, who was then eight, turned to his father and pointed at me, saying, "Dad, why is Mom all red?"

I was able to suppress the reaction enough to complete the holiday and continue with the chemotherapy, but as I did each treatment the possibility that the next one would trigger a lethal allergic reaction grew stronger. Faced with the likelihood that I was now risking death in order to cheat it, I stopped.

The fact that I could not easily clear the toxic chemotherapy from my body led me to wonder if I had also struggled to clear toxins I had been exposed to in my hometown. My sister, Sue, had struggled mightily with her chemotherapy as well.

I knew scientists were studying the heritable variations in our susceptibility to environmental agents and I wondered if more than others, my sister and I lacked some ability to eliminate toxins from our bodies. After all, there is a range of human reaction to all manner of beneficial and harmful substances.

There is no way to know if I did enough chemotherapy for it to make a difference; no way to know if my decision to do the chemotherapy was the right one at all. If my cancer does not come back, it may be because I was completely cured by surgery, or it may be that the drugs killed whatever cancerous cells were left. If it does come back, it may mean that the drugs had no effect, or it may mean that the drugs significantly slowed the return of the disease. I will just never know. Ever.

CHAPTER TEN

Destiny

CANCER SURVIVORS ARE supposed to be new, shiny versions of their former selves—more spiritually aware, slightly more alive, and a bit more grateful for everything. In the parlance of those who study illness and people's reactions to it, this is a "restitution narrative."[1] You've gotten your life back, you've garnered important spiritual and personal lessons, and you've put the experience behind you.

It's a hard line to walk, and I did a pretty poor job of it. I wasn't better; I was just more creaky and a lot more cranky. I did, however, experience renewal in one sense. I had a renewed desire to complete what I had started for my sister. Only this time it was about me too.

Back at the hospital where I was treated, I signed up for a second round of genetic testing. This time my geneticist was a dark-haired woman with multiple degrees and a name with so many consonants that I skipped trying to pronounce it. She reviewed my charts and looked at my family tree with its boxes and circles.

She then correctly surmised that the commercially

available tests would reveal no known genetic key to unlock the mysteries of my disease, my sister's, or their relationship—our cancers were too rare and there were too few incidences within our family. We went through the motions one more time anyhow. Three small tubes of my blood were packed in bubble wrap and sent in a small box to a lab in Utah. When the results came back with no known genetic mutations, I was disappointed but not surprised.

The author Alice Munro once wrote, "There is no protection unless it is in knowing. I wanted to know. I wanted death pinned down and isolated behind a wall of particular facts and circumstances, not floating around loose, ignored, but powerful, waiting to get in anywhere."[2]

I wanted to know too. I wanted to know more about what role the pollutants in Lake Michigan might have played in our cancers and what role our genes could have played as well. It's a common misconception to think that cancer is "caused" by either genes or environment. Instead, a kind of dance between genes and the environment, with each one influencing the other, is what leads to disease. By the time I was diagnosed, my sister had a granddaughter and my son was eight years old. We had passed one copy of our genes to our children, and we had also passed along our chemical body burdens—years of stored exposures—as we carried our children within us and then breastfed them.

There are elaborate systems for diagnosing and treating disease, but there is no system that easily helps people think about the cause of a serious illness like cancer. Doctors in many cases tend to dismiss its origin as irrelevant or unknowable. Geneticists are more sympathetic, but their knowledge is limited to diseases that clearly run in families and to what can be gleaned using a few genetic tests. Toxicologists know in-depth the effects of certain chemicals, but without knowing the amount and timing of an exposure, in addition to possible exposures to other chemicals, they can't say much.

Even knowing how to ask fruitful questions about the origins of your disease and its possible links with certain chemicals is challenging. Each of us carries a lifetime of chemical exposures that we squire around with us each day. Some of these chemicals persist in our body for decades, and some of them are passed on from generation to generation.

While scientists once followed the centuries-old rubric that "the dose makes the poison" and focused on determining effects at high levels of exposure, a new science is emerging that looks at the consequences of the low doses that virtually all of us store in our bodies. "The new science of low dose exposure is challenging centuries of accepted wisdom about toxic substances," heralded the *Wall Street Journal* in a 2005 front-page article. "Using advanced lab techniques, scientists have found that with some chemicals, traces as minute as mere parts per trillion have biological effects. With some of these chemicals, such trace levels exist in the blood and urine of the general population."3

Making matters more complicated, chemicals can have one effect at a small dose and a different effect or no effect at all at a higher dose. Similarly, some chemicals have greater effects when found in combination with other chemicals—a situation familiar to anyone who has ever mixed several kinds of alcohol in one night and suffered the results. Some chemicals may simply fuel growth in a cancer that already exists, as environmental estrogens are believed to do. There is evidence that certain chemicals, such as PCBs, lower immune function, making it that much easier to develop a disease. And some chemicals may actually change the way our bodies rid themselves of toxins, so that one dose of a toxin makes us that much more vulnerable to the next. As such, many of these chemicals are thought to promote disease, as opposed to actually "causing" it in the way that a virus causes the flu.

Finally, our various genetic makeups may make us more or less susceptible to cancer-causing chemicals or other toxins. Just as we all have different tolerances for different medicines, we may have different tolerances for different toxic exposures. In one study, for example, scientists at first could find no relationship between breast cancer and PCB levels in the women who suffered from the disease. However, when researchers selected a group of women out of the main study who shared a specific gene variant that made it difficult for them to clear toxins from their bodies, a more significant relationship was discovered.[4]

"Cancer," writes Stanford professor Robert Proctor, "can be understood as a consequence of defects in genetic regulation, but also as a result of environmental insults. There are proximate and ultimate causes of cancer, biological and social causes, and a focus on the one need not preclude a focus on the other."[5]

Scientists often scoff at suggestions that any one thing, by itself, "causes" cancer—and for good reason, given the many processes involved. At a minimum two things need to happen in order for a cancer to form. A tumor-suppressor gene, which restrains a cell's ability to divide, must be knocked out; and a growth-promoter gene, called an oncogene, must be turned on. These two changes allow the cell to go on its growth rampage. The increasing rate of cell division in such a rampage means an increased chance of further mutations and a greater chance with each mutation for a higher degree of malignancy.[6]

These changes have been demonstrated over and over again by using what are called knock-out mice. By manipulating, or knocking out, the particular genes of lab mice, scientists are able to create disease and thereby tease out the role of each gene in the process. Daniela Dinulescu, a Romanian researcher at MIT, created the first mouse model of ovarian cancer in 2004. By taking a healthy mouse and activating an oncogene known as KRAS, Dinulescu was first able to create a mouse with endometriosis. When she then knocked out both copies of a tumor-suppressor gene called PTEN, the mouse also developed ovarian cancer.

While this kind of process is painfully clear in the lab, it is less clear in humans. Scientists do not know what starts the tumble of genetic changes necessary to cause disease. It could be a substance, it could be a virus, it could be a simple error in the reproduction of a cell. In some cases, the answer is clear: sunlight, asbestos, cigarette smoke. In other cases, like my own and my sister's, the answer is less so.

Individuals inherit genes from their parents, but except in the case of rare, clearly inherited illnesses such as Huntington's, diseases themselves are not passed down. Genes do not confer a preordained destiny. Our lives and our health are the outcome of our own genetic predispositions intertwined with our environment, including what we eat, drink, breathe, and touch. This is what scientists call the genes-times-environment equation, or GxE. There is a saying in the field: "Genetics loads the gun; environment pulls the trigger."[7]

Toxic chemicals can play two important roles in cancer causation. They can either start the process by creating the original mutations, or they can supply excess estrogen to feed aberrant growths that already exist—thereby promoting cancer's spread. As such, the environment can either help to start the process or can promote it once it has begun.

To demonstrate this point, researchers from the University of Pittsburgh Cancer Institute's Center for Environmental Oncology recently took fish that were heavily contaminated with endocrine-disrupting chemicals from the polluted nearby Monongahela River and distilled them into a liquid extract using a special solvent. When they fed the liquefied fish to a strain of breast cancer cells called MCF-7, the cells grew quickly. "We used this cell line, MCF-7, because it has estrogen receptors in it, meaning that if estrogens are present it causes the cell line to proliferate," says Conrad Volz, codirector of exposure assessment at the cancer institute. "If you put something on it and it grows, then it must be stimulating the estrogen receptor."[8] In this case, the pollutants in the fish were literally causing the breast cancer cells to grow.

Studying the medical histories of immigrants can also shed light on the relationship between the environment and disease. Throughout the last century, women in Japan had much lower rates of breast cancer than women in the United States. But women of Japanese descent whose ancestors moved to the United States two or three generations earlier exhibit breast cancer rates much closer to the American average. "Clearly, environmental differences account for the difference in cancer rates," says Bill Thilly, director of MIT's Center for Environmental Health Sciences.[9] Whatever genetic possibilities for developing breast cancer the women carried, they were jolted awake by something encountered in the United States, whether a variation in diet, lifestyle, or exposure to new levels of toxins.

Epigenetics, or the study of how the environment may awaken sleeping genetic possibilities in certain populations such as in the example above, is emerging as a new paradigm in cancer research. "Genetic predispositions may have once been just that, inclinations never fulfilled," writes James Olson in *Bathsheba's Breast*. "But after the Industrial Revolution, dormant genetic impulses may have become transfigured into deadly imperatives, awakened by modern chemistry and rapid social change."[10]

Stark examples of this can be found in rapidly industrializing China, where according to *China Daily* the incidence of many different kinds of cancer is rising. The people of China have now won what each and every American claims as a birthright: an exposure to a chemical cocktail of air pollutants, water pollutants, and pesticides in food. Overall, cancer incidence rates in China have gone up 4.2 percent per year, but pancreatic cancer cases are skyrocketing. One hospital reported a sixfold increase in pancreatic cancer patients since the mid-1950s.[11]

Pancreatic cancer, in general, suffers from a dearth of funding relative to other deadly cancers. And the number of full-time researchers studying the disease is small, so little is known about its origins—in China or elsewhere.[12] One study that has been published, though, looked at 108 cases of pancreatic cancer and 82 controls for differences in blood levels of PCBs. Those who had the highest levels of PCBs in their blood were more than four times as likely as the controls to have pancreatic cancer—a small but striking study.[13]

☙

A few years ago, I made a trip to the registry of pancreatic cancer tumors at Johns Hopkins University. I wanted to register my tumor, which was remarkable because it was a rare form of the cancer, not because it was a large tumor—amazingly enough, there have been bigger ones.

At Johns Hopkins each patient is given a small card with a bar code, and you check yourself in—sort of the way you let yourself into a health club or an office. On this day, I carried my slides and a large piece of film that showed my insides with the tumor intact. I was directed down several hallways, leaving the fish tanks and the fancy furniture for halls that looked like an old high school, with bright lights and lockers lining the sides. I was in the pathology department—a place most patients never see—where tumors are scored and fates decided.

I knocked at the door of a well-known pathologist and began to recite my health history. About 1,500 people have registered their tumors. Of these, about 600 have more than one family member with the disease—most notably, President Jimmy Carter, whose father, brother, and both sisters died of the disease.

I was five minutes into my story when the pathologist stopped me. "I know your story," he said, pulling a copy of my slides out of a file on his desk. "I teach your case."

I imagined myself as a trick question on some pathology test, but he assured me not. I have a rare cancer and it is helpful for young pathologists to see it, that's all. Over the course of a long career, pathologists must develop the ability to note small differences in the appearances of cells. In order to develop this intense pattern recognition, they must see hundreds upon hundreds of slides. Showing me my slides, the pathologist told me a few facts about my disease.

What he did not do, despite my badgering, was tell me what he thinks led to my disease. Few doctors ever do that.

We chatted briefly and politely. Smoking is the biggest risk factor for pancreatic cancer, he said. Neither my sister nor I smoked, but like many in our generation, we inhaled a ton of secondhand smoke at home because both our parents were smokers.

The pathologist told me that President Carter has drawn attention to the field because of the depth of the disease in his family and because, well, he was president. Carter narrated a public-service ad about the disease not long ago. Some have questioned whether the Carter family's exposures to agricultural pesticides or herbicides on the family peanut farm played a role in the disease. Moreover, nuts can carry a natural carcinogen called aflatoxin.

Then the pathologist told me one more important fact. My particular form of pancreatic cancer occurs more frequently in women by a ratio of 9 to 1.[14] This holds true for mucinous cystadenocarcinomas (MCACs) of other organs, including of the appendix and the biliary system.

I was impressed by the overwhelming predominance of women who develop my disease, and when I returned to Boston I decided to investigate. While I did not develop an ovarian cancer like my sister's, I definitely developed a woman's disease. And there are similarities between my disease and certain kinds of ovarian cancer.

Like true ovarian tissues, the tissue samples from tumors like my own contain estrogen receptors. According to a paper on 130 pancreatic MCAC cases at Johns Hopkins, only tumors removed from women demonstrate a tissue structure similar to that found in ovarian cells.[15] To me, these numbers imply that estrogen or other female-specific hormones could be involved in the tumor-generation process, and that means that chemicals in Lake Michigan that act as artificial estrogens could indeed be a critical factor.

Furthermore, cells taken from mucinous tumors show mucin production patterns that respond to the introduction of an estrogen mimic—such as the chemicals found in my hometown. Thus, estrogen, and possibly artificial estrogens of the type that lined the lake, may preferentially promote the growth of MCAC in women.

I tried to explain this to my gynecologist in Boston while undergoing a routine exam. He listened respectfully enough, then shrugged. He had helped me through my pregnancy, and he knew the details of my sister's death and my pain surrounding it. He had ordered many of my routine screenings before my cancer took hold. He had weighed in during my decision to do chemotherapy.

"Look, Nancy," he said, "I don't know what caused your cancer or your sister's cancer, but whatever it was, it got you. Either the genes or the exposures or both."

For this doctor, on that day, there was no reason to parse things too finely. You have it, or you don't. Who cares what caused it? In coping with the immediate needs of his patients, this approach works. It's not my doctor's job to ponder the possibilities; he must see to my safety. But on another level, society loses out when we ignore the cause to look for the cure.

The pressing issue of cause and effect lay before me, however. That is, I still had my ovaries and they continued to be a risk. This doctor, along with many others, believed I should have them taken out.

⌒⟫

"Destiny, Mom. Destiny!" My son is screaming this from inside the house. I am out on the deck, reading and rereading the first twenty-four pages of a slim novel he has been reading at school. A fourth-grade teacher has assigned *destiny* as a vocabulary word, and he must find it in the text and then derive its meaning from the context. No luck, however. The word is not on the page the teacher suggested, nor on any other page near it. I am convinced there is a mistake on the worksheet she has given him. My son, however, who believes this teacher cannot fail in any way—ever—is not ready to give up.

The phone rings. A friend is calling to tell me that a woman from our book club has died of ovarian cancer. She is the third person to tell me this in twenty-four hours, and each time I hear it I retreat to my bedroom to cry—for the woman who died, for her children, for my sister, for me, and for no reason at all, since I have finally decided to have my ovaries removed.

When I was finally ready to make this decision, the choice was among the easiest I encountered in my long medical odyssey, and it was one of the few that generated anything close to consensus among my physicians. If Nike hadn't owned the phrase "Just Do It," I believe my doctors would have patented it. Their thinking was uniform.

I had given birth to my child and would not have another. Further, my ability to develop one cancer may have put me at risk for developing others. While genetic testing had not turned up any specific indicator of disease, the relative similarity of my sister's tumors to mine had raised an eyebrow or two. The dance between my genes and my environmental exposures, my own GxE, had turned into a heated flamenco. Destiny might be too strong a word for it, but it was the one my son had ringing in my head. As one doctor reasonably said, "What's the point of beating pancreatic cancer and then dying of ovarian cancer?" To that argument, I had no answer.

Any woman who has ever doubted the power of estrogen, whether the bucket loads of it in your body when you are young or the minute amounts encountered regularly in environmental exposures, ought to try ripping her ovaries out. Surgical menopause can be more intense than regular menopause, and my experience was no exception. I sweated through pajamas night after night. I had mood swings so severe that I was in danger of wrecking my marriage. Sex became so painful that I endured weeks of physical therapy simply to be able to attempt it again. Eventually, I washed up on the other side of this major transition. I was less sexy, I was less strong, my skin had lost any semblance of tightness, but I was alive, a survivor.

CHAPTER ELEVEN

Why Ask Why?

Survivorship has its own rewards: Christmas, ski trips, the chance to see your kid in the play, to write another story, to watch TV while your husband falls asleep in his chair. To have that occasional good run or fast swim that makes you think you might eventually feel normal someday.

Survivorship also comes with its own expectations: to look as good as you can, to be upbeat and not too morbid, and, most importantly, to not ask too many questions about the cause of your cancer. To not push too hard against that heavy internal resistance to looking, really looking, at what we might be doing to the world around us and what it in turn might be doing to us.

What you choose to tell yourself about your illness or a family member's illness can affect how you experience it, how you choose to fight it, and even how you conjure it up as memory. The stories we tell ourselves about our experiences are often as potent as the experiences themselves.

At a societal level, the way we talk and think about disease is critical, too. When we talk only about the risks of toxic chemicals, for instance, instead of about the known harms associated with chemicals we all encounter every day, we create both a false uncertainty and a roadblock for reforms that could reduce the levels of toxins in children and adults alike.

Though the recent movement to brand cancer patients as "survivors" has bred a welcome sense of hope and optimism for many, it has also helped blind us to the vast environmental changes that have wracked our world and our bodies.

When I asked a young graduate student who helped me research this book why she had chosen the field of public health, she told me this parable: "If you see a baby floating down the river, you save it, you don't ask, Why is this baby here? But when there are thousands of babies floating down the river and you can't save them all anymore, then you have to ask, What's up with the babies in the river? Where are they coming from?"

She is right: We have to stop to ask. Asking saved my life. Asking the larger questions will help save the lives of others. But asking, however, is at present a radical and not uniformly accepted idea. Most people believe it is better not to waste time wondering why and instead marshal resources to cope with disease when it strikes.

In February 2007 an article appeared in the *Boston Globe* about a man whose wife had pancreatic cancer. This couple lived less than half a mile from a well-known Massachusetts Superfund site, in a community with high rates of cancer. Cancer clusters are very hard to verify, but in this case the state did not hesitate to identify those living closest to the site as having unusually high rates of cancer. In fact, that story had been splashed across the front pages of the *Globe* weeks earlier. Yet in this later story about the man and his wife, the writer downplayed the couple's proximity to the Superfund site and instead wrote that the man needed to "relinquish his anger and accept what he can't change." The man did this, the writer celebrated, by jumping into a local, frigid reservoir in what the headline called an "affirming ritual."[1]

The writer did not suggest that this man should dwell on the cause of his wife's cancer, become politically active, and try to save others from his wife's fate. Asking why, or in this case knowing why and getting angry about it, does not fit the modern-day survivor narrative. Somehow, jumping into a cold reservoir in winter makes sense; asking why does not.

The *Boston Globe* is not alone in repeating this theme. The large cancer centers in our country print glossy magazines to promote their services, herald their research, and tell their success stories, all the while soliciting donations. Since I have been treated at several of these institutions, I receive several different magazines. All of them trumpet the no-holds-barred cancer patient who never stops to ask why and never stops fighting his or her personal disease.

A 2006 issue makes this point clearly. "The unexpected news that Tom's cancer had returned was even harder to take. Though the timing couldn't have been worse for the couple, Tom and Nicole chose not to torture themselves with the unanswerable 'why us' and 'why now?' Instead they devoted their energy to fighting the recurrence."[2]

This attitude—this don't ask, don't wonder, don't stop even to consider why—is in part a form of self-protection. Searching for causes risks the possibility of self-blaming. Some popular writers, for instance, have promoted the idea that there is a cancer personality or that those whose cancers return somehow wished it upon themselves. I am certainly not advocating a blame-the-victim view. I am not even against jumping into a cold reservoir if it makes you feel better. I am against us all collectively pretending that we can't know what causes our cancers or that the causes are of only minor importance. What I am getting at is what psychiatrists call our "selective inattention to detail," the ability to create an atmosphere in which people can ignore an inconvenient reality—that, say, your mother is an alcoholic or that the way we are living, consuming, and polluting is pathological.

Such distortion happens on the scientific front as well. Just as we create knowledge and scientific advances, we also create ignorance. Industries have become vastly effective at sponsoring studies that support their point of view, while controversies are made to drag on for decades before they are resolved—if they are ever resolved at all. As the tobacco companies were bold enough to say: doubt is our product. This strategy has served industry well for decades.

Robert Proctor calls this the social construction of ignorance. "The persistence of controversy is often not a natural consequence of imperfect knowledge," he writes, "but a political consequence of conflicting interests and structural apathies. Controversy can be engineered; ignorance and uncertainty can be manufactured, maintained, and disseminated."[3] Not asking why has its benefits, certainly, for those who pollute; and that is part of the price we pay for the mythology we are weaving around the idea of survivorship.

While it may make sense—certainly does make sense—for any given person to decide that he or she will not, cannot, should not ask why, we lose something as a society when legions of survivors make the same choice. Hundreds of individuals making the right choices for themselves may be making the wrong choice for society as a whole. Economists call this problem the tragedy of the commons. The tragedy is that no individual has the means or the incentive to do what must be done for the future of society as a whole. Instead, each jumps into the lake and hopes for the best.

During the summer I was sick with chemo, Lance Armstrong won the Tour de France. I watched him race, his sinewy legs pumping, pumping, his inspirational almost unbelievable comeback story flashing across the screen.

As I lay there on the couch in a chemo-induced haze, he represented an almost unimaginable return to health and vitality. Often during chemotherapy I had bouts of unbearable fatigue. We used to call them "Mama's been hit by the bus days." Often I felt that I wouldn't be able to get up even if the house were on fire.

So I lay there watching Lance, hoping he wouldn't fall, hoping some crazed fan wouldn't drag him off his bike, knowing that hundreds of people were, like me, in treatment during this week, many of them watching him climb higher and higher—pinning their hopes of survival on him as he rode over cobblestones and up precarious mountain paths, swerving around fallen riders and roadside obstacles. He may have been as vulnerable, maybe even more vulnerable, than we were. I watched him tackle the route day after day on his rail-thin lightweight bike. I said to myself, "See, if he can do it, I can too." Or worse, other people said to me, "See, if he can do it, you can too."

That fall I visited Washington, DC, with my husband and son over Columbus Day weekend and watched Lance finish a cross-country ride sponsored by the drug company that had made the chemo that saved him. I stood on the mall where as a nation we have memorialized all our warriors—those from the great world wars that united us and those from the divisive Vietnam War. As Lance rode victorious into our nation's capital with a peloton of other cancer survivors who rode with him, the streets were lined with those who also wore the winner's yellow jersey—those who had won their own personal battles with cancer.

He was glistening with sweat and stunning, with his zero percent body fat and his legacy of surviving, not just a difficult childhood, but a cancer that at the time was one of the deadliest. The symbolism was clear: he was a warrior returned victorious from the worst kind of battle, a rock-star survivor who had made it back from the other side, and so, by inference, were the others. He had survived, they had survived, and now we were all together celebrating. See, this cancer thing, this chemo thing, no big problem.

This spectacle of the victorious warrior reinforces the cultural perception of what battling cancer is all about. There are, after all, legions of cancer survivors, diagnosed but not dead. Cured maybe, or maybe in remission. We have all been to the other side. We are marked by the burns on our skin that the chemo left as it coursed through our veins, or, in my own case, marked with a ten-inch scar across my abdomen.

My son was eight when I was diagnosed. I spent many months hiding my scar from him. We were at a hotel in the Berkshires during one of my treatment weeks. I went to the room to change into my swimsuit. He was playing on the other side of the room, and my back was to him as I changed. Then, from outside the room I heard a loud bang. Instinctually, I turned to check on my son. He, too, turned to me. And I stood fully exposed to him for the first time since my surgery.

He took one long look at my scar and dropped into a fighting stance known on battlefields and playgrounds worldwide—arms outstretched, fists clenched.

"Ooooo, Mama Warrior," he said. "She just battles through the pain."

He was not simply reacting to his sick mother, who rallied to drive him to soccer, to baseball, to the doctor; who, throwing up and clearly experiencing intense vertigo, still came when the school called to say he'd been kicked too hard with a soccer ball. In his short, sweet gesture, he was acknowledging and reinforcing a broad cultural perception that folks with my disease fight it. Individuals battle cancer and, as a society, we have been fighting a great war against cancer—our very own medical Vietnam, as one physician called it, but a war nonetheless.

Standing on the mall in Washington I knew I was a warrior of sorts, but I wasn't sure I would emerge victorious. And I was too close to my own treatment to believe that coping with chemotherapy was no big deal. I certainly wasn't ready to don the yellow jersey, but I was hoping that someday I would be able to.

Yet I found it hard not to be affected by the cultural significance of this gathering. Lance was every bit as much a hero as the generals of yesteryear. Cancer was not a disease to be ashamed of, but somehow something to be proud of— with survivors being treated like rock stars. Standing among the crowd, my young son at my side, I was struck by how much attitudes had changed over the preceding thirty years.

I can recall being a child and hearing about women who were sick with cancer. You were at the grocery store or the library or out for a stroll when you heard that so and so had gone in for an operation, and the surgeons had taken one look and simply closed her back up. Doctors have a phrase for such operations; they call them "peek and shriek" surgeries. You didn't even name the disease back then, and, if you were forced to, you had to whisper it.

But all of that has changed. A relative I see only rarely recently visited me and announced in my kitchen most proudly that she had metastatic cancer. How did we go from the disease that cannot be named to the disease that makes you a superstar? The status comes complete with walks, and rides, and ribbons, and yellow jerseys that prove you have not only been tested, but have endured, maybe even conquered.

There is a fashion to sickness. Illness, after all, unless you happen to have it, is simply an idea—and ideas can be manipulated. In *Illness as Metaphor*, Susan Sontag charts the social history of two diseases—tuberculosis and cancer. Sontag tells us that despite its horrific manifestations, tuberculosis was widely romanticized at the end of the 1800s and well into the 1900s. Those with tuberculosis were seen as passionate, with galloping ardor and unusual powers of seduction. Their disease was dubbed "consumption," since it was believed to consume all that was negative or dirty—leaving only the patients' white shining souls and the incomparable beauty bestowed by their illness.

Not so, cancer. At the time Sontag was writing, and was diagnosed herself, cancer continued to bear a sizable stigma. Writing in 1977—a mere thirty years ago—Sontag called cancer "a disease that nobody has managed to glamorize."[4] Historically, cancer had been associated with the stench of decaying flesh and the screaming of those forced to endure a painful death.

Breast cancer, in particular, was a source of shame and a disease that you hid. It wasn't until Betty Ford and

Happy Rockefeller, the wives of the president and vice president, respectively, went public with their back-to-back mastectomies in the fall of 1974 that the stigma began to subside. Two years later, in 1976, New York newswoman Betty Rollin wrote a bestselling book—later made into a popular television movie—about her own breast cancer called *First, You Cry*.

Rollin's book may have been the first popular breast cancer narrative, but it was not the last. Breast cancer has come out of the closet, and the idea of survivorship has even become sexy. In *Why I Wore Lipstick to My Mastectomy*, the author recounts going to a strip club before her surgery to understand the power of breasts and to make her medical decisions while in what she calls mammary mecca. In the television movie derived from the book, the stripper scene translates powerfully. Similarly, in the graphic novel *Cancer Vixen*, the heroine wears stilettos to her chemo, while claiming, "Cancer, I am going to kick your butt, and I am going to do it in killer five inch heels."[5]

While the steep decline in stigmatization of cancer patients is a great boon, particularly for women, there is a dark side to the ascendancy of cancer patients as rock stars, as lipstick-wearing kick-ass survivors. The medical sociologist and cancer survivor Arthur Frank says with the wisdom of one who has been there that this Phoenix rising from the ashes metaphor, this ability to come out stronger and wiser, is a liberation, but a burden too. And there is a very specific dark side for many individuals: are those who don't survive failures?

One has to ask, why this incredible cultural shift in just thirty years? Certainly there have been advances, and those must be applauded. But the war has yet to be won, even if there have been successful battles and a few warriors have returned safely—gloriously so in Lance's case.

If cancer patients are the new rock stars, if the popular image of cancer patients is of us jubilant on a walkathon, conquering our disease, or at least raising money to someday conquer it, folks don't have to see us in the other way—curled up on the bathroom floor waiting for the antinausea medicine to kick in, lining up to get the IV drip, nursing our wounds from surgery, watching our hair go down the drain with our vitality and our sexuality and taking with it our dignity, our jobs, and sometimes even our marriages.

If we keep warring, winning, and walking, we and others around us don't have to stop and ask: What made her sick? What the hell is happening to my mother, my sister, that nice lady down the street? Because the common belief is that this disease is now conquerable—maybe not in every case, but look at Lance, look at all those women with the bald heads and the pink baseball caps smiling. That's success. And there have been amazing advances indeed—especially in the disease Lance had, testicular cancer.

And yet, without taking anything away from the curable cases, the amazing advances, the spirit of those willing to walk for three days straight or bicycle across the country, the superstar cancer-patient image is simply a new kind of invisibility. It denies, or at least downplays, the suffering that comes with the disease and in doing so makes it easier to avoid thinking too hard about the causes. As Arthur Frank writes in his beautiful book *At the Will of the Body*, "The fault and the fear are safely contained, locked up inside the cancer patient. Cigarette companies can stay in business, polluters can pollute, advertisers can glorify sunbathing, and those who enjoy good health can believe they have earned it."[6]

It is, after all, so much easier to think of Lance as the courageous survivor, even victor that he is, rather than to think about what could have made the rate of testicular cancer triple between 1940 and 1980—post–World War II years when the use of toxic chemicals in our society blossomed.7

"I have no quarrel with the notion of survivors, but my first choice as a designation is witness," Frank says. Witnesses give testimony, and "testimony implicates others in what they witness."8 So how about this: what if, instead of calling me a cancer survivor, people just looked at me and said, look at that gray-haired lady, there goes another woman who was a victim of industrial pollution. She is a reminder that we need to rethink the products we buy, the way they are produced, and how they are disposed of. That would certainly change the equation, wouldn't it?

For me, being a survivor is not good enough. I don't simply want to outlive my disease. I want to live my life with meaning, and for that I have one powerful role model. In the annals of environmental history no testimony has been as effective as that of Rachel Carson. Soon after *Silent Spring* was published in 1962, Carson testified before Congress, and her testimony led to the banning of DDT and helped set in motion the modern environmental movement.

What few people know is that Carson struggled with breast cancer while writing the powerful chapters that linked DDT to human disease. If the words *cancer causing* and *chemical* have become inseparable in the minds of many Americans, we have Carson to thank.

Carson chose not to make her cancer public at the time, instead encouraging her friends to tell people that she never looked better. And although Carson never directly related her disease to chemical exposure, a few notes in her letters to her dear friend Dorothy Freeman make it appear that she at least worried about a connection. "Of course, one should also make a strong effort to eliminate the chlorinated hydrocarbons from one's own food," she wrote. "But civilization has made it so very difficult to do that!"9

Carson died in 1964, but her work and her life serve as a warning to everyone who struggles with cancer. "As we pour our millions into research and invest all our hopes in vast programs to find cures for established cases of cancer," she wrote, "we are neglecting the golden opportunity to prevent, even while we seek to cure."10

Carson's favorite quote, from Abraham Lincoln, can be found snuggled into her almost daily letters to Freeman, where she explains what keeps her going through her treatments and on to finish her groundbreaking book. It reads: "To sin by silence when they should protest, makes cowards of men."11

CHAPTER TWELVE

Proof

Cᴀɴ ʏᴏᴜ ᴘʀᴏᴠᴇ ᴛʜᴀᴛ these chemicals caused either your sister's or your cancer? I mean, really, can you prove this?" My husband is standing behind the kitchen counter. We are cleaning up before bed, wiping the counters and picking up stray bits of food off the floor. He is tired of this project, my cancer, and me—all at the same time. The idea of cancer survivor as witness is all well and good, but right now I am failing.

I would blow off his comment and attribute it to late-night crankiness or the inevitable stress of knowing your spouse has a potentially fatal disease if not for one thing. My husband is a former federal prosecutor with many years experience prosecuting environmental crimes. He knows what it takes to prove that these chemicals are dangerous—at least in court. Somewhere between my sister's diagnosis and my own, he had settled a $2.5 million case against a large company for dumping contaminated waste oils into the Charles River near Harvard Square.

My husband understands at a very basic level how the everyday decisions of managers—not to fix that leak or comply with that one ornery regulation—can end up turn-ing into a decades-long environmental nightmare. In the case of my illness, however, it is his personal nightmare. The faraway environmental woes of Waukegan, Illinois, have come to fruition in his house in Boston and are currently staring him down over the kitchen counter.

His question, and the curt way he delivers it, stops me short. I take a quick breath. Our eyes lock. "So, can you?" he says, the way a schoolboy would taunt a playmate.

I withered under his kitchen cross-examination that night, shuffling off to bed without answering. Weeks later, I have finally come up with the answer I should have given him. The French have a saying for this: *l'esprit de l'escalier*—literally, the wit of the staircase—the preferable, pointed response that would have proven one's superiority had it not come to mind too late.

What I now understand that I didn't fully grasp before my little kitchen confrontation is that there are different standards for proof depending on the venue. There is the legal standard of proof—complete with what counts as evi-dence and whose testimony matters—that my husband knows all too well. Then there is the scientific standard, and that also comes with its own set of rules—including publi-cation in a journal where your peers decide if your research is acceptable. And then, in the context of public safety, there is the kind of proof that regulators depend on to decide whether or not they should act. How do you know that some-thing is dangerous enough to ban it? What are the costs and what are the benefits of regulation? Finally, there is that per-sonal moment when you yourself become convinced of one thing or another, when you finally "know" something in such a way that you cannot simply forget it or imagine it not to be true. Our discourse around modern chemicals and the environment and health are often a jumble of all these.

For starters, let's look at the legal requirements for proof. What my husband understood at an intimate level would astound me when I later cracked open the law books. The courts' distinct mandate to mete out justice means that they must have a specific standard of proof and a specific standard of evidence, especially with respect to scientific evidence. Not only could I not prove in a courtroom setting that these chemicals caused my cancer, much of the evidence I have marshaled in this book would not even be admissible in court.[1]

My argument is not a simple or a straightforward one. There is no smoking gun. There is no perfect study to prove that the chemicals in Lake Michigan contributed to, or caused, or promoted my disease or my sister's. Instead, I have made an extended argument that rests on the weight of the evidence in its entirety—the way the oil dripped into the troughs in the factories, the way the sands in the lake shifted in the harbor, the ugly discards at the landfill, animal studies, chemical analyses of the blood of humans across the nation, the effects of various chemicals on fish and other wildlife, the exact nature of cellular changes when cancer cells are fed certain chemical substances—all sorts of data pieced together in an elaborate web.

But this does not meet my husband's legal standard. Indeed, he pointed out a relevant case to help me understand why my case would be most difficult to get into a courtroom.

Robert Joiner was an electrician in the Water and Light Department in Thomasville, Georgia. He worked with and around electrical transformers manufactured by General

Electric (GE), some of which held fluids that contained PCBs, furans, or dioxins. In order to repair the transformers, Joiner often had to stick his hands into the fluid, and he claimed that the fluid had also sometimes splashed into his eyes and mouth. Many years after his exposure, Joiner—who had also smoked for eight years—contracted lung cancer, a disease some of his relatives had also had. He sued GE in Georgia's state court, claiming that his exposure to PCBs had "promoted" his cancer.

GE's lawyers petitioned successfully to move the case to federal court, where the standard of harm and the standards for introducing evidence would be more favorable to their case. They then immediately asked that the case be dismissed on the grounds that there was no admissible scientific evidence that PCBs had promoted Joiner's cancer.

Joiner's lawyers responded by making an argument not dissimilar to the one I am making in this book. Citing the work of at least thirteen different researchers and the reports of the World Health Organization, they extrapolated from animal studies and occupational studies to show that Joiner's exposure to PCBs, dioxins, and furans may have played a significant role in his cancer, even if they were not the sole cause of his disease.

The U.S. District Court in Georgia ruled in favor of the manufacturer, rejecting the expert testimony of the plaintiffs as "subjective belief or unsupported speculation" and ruling it inadmissible.[2] Joiner's case was in legal terms, *ipse dixit*, an assertion made but not proven—based as much, or more, on the authority of experts and the force of their arguments than on the power of the evidence marshaled.

The U.S. Court of Appeals briefly reinstated the testimony, but the Supreme Court ruled in favor of the manufacturer in 1997, arguing that the studies Joiner and his team of experts used were not relevant. Justice Stevens, in the minority, disagreed. Noting that the U.S. Environmental Protection Agency uses methods similar to Joiner's experts when deciding on regulations, Justice Stevens wrote, "It is not intrinsically 'unscientific' for experienced professionals to arrive at a conclusion by weighing all available scientific evidence."[3]

Still, the view of the majority held, and a new standard had been set. In the years since the ruling in *General Electric v. Joiner* and rulings in several related cases, it has become progressively more difficult to pursue courtroom remedies in the face of chemical contamination. Stringent rules of evidence have effectively prevented cases against all kinds of dangerous substances—most notably tobacco, Agent Orange, and asbestos—from advancing in the courts.[4]

I lament this fact to my husband on one of our many dates that have turned into mini legal classes for me and a big drag for him. "Bad facts make bad law," I say, explaining yet again why I think my own case is a stronger one than Joiner's. My case is not complicated by cigarette smoking. Our understanding of cancer and the way that it develops is now much more nuanced than it was at the time of Joiner's trial. I go on at length, giving my husband little respite.

He gives me the polite smile of a husband who knows he must spend the rest of his life with his wife, and surely there is no reason to pick a fight with someone as intent as I am—certainly he has nothing to gain, even though we both know that I am not quite meeting his courtroom test. The bar is so high, the standards so tough, it is next to impossible to make a case that might hold up in the courtroom.

My argument, like Joiner's case, is based on the weight

of scientific evidence, the presence of the chemicals in my hometown, and the many ways my sister and I might have been exposed. Still, the implications of my failure to mount a courtroom-worthy argument are enormous. Not only have arguments like my own and Joiner's and hundreds of others faced increasingly difficult hurdles in the legal system, the very nuanced way in which these chemicals affect our bodies at such low levels means that regulation, too, has become increasingly more difficult to pursue. It is ironic, to say the least, that as more and more evidence has come to light, proving causality in an airtight, lockstep, linear way has become ever more difficult. My situation is a thoroughly modern one. I have no courtroom-worthy proof, and yet I have no reason to doubt either.

It is nearly impossible to prove that a particular person's cancer results from a particular chemical, at least in terms of the standards of legal proof. It is also difficult to determine, within the limits of scientific inquiry, whether a particular individual's cancer results from a particular chemical exposure. As a rule, scientists dislike the word *proof*, avoiding it the way most people avoid poison ivy. Ask a scientist for proof and you will likely get lectured on how it is impossible to conclusively prove anything. Any scientist who claims to have "proof" of anything, or complains that "there is no proof," is likely to generate suspicion among his or her peers. Instead, scientists prefer to work in groups that refer to a body of scientific evidence and that cite the plausibility, strength, and consistency of causal associations when supporting or rejecting a particular claim.

Like a jury, groups exploring a given scientific question, such as "does this chemical cause cancer" or "what exposure level is safe," typically work by consensus, weighing, rating, and arguing over the evidence and crafting evidence-based statements to argue over some more. When they are through, all must agree with the committee's conclusions and statements before any findings can be published.

When it comes to cancer, exposure, and "proof," the International Agency for Research on Cancer (IARC) is the premier organization for evidence-based science. The IARC is funded and administered by the United Nations as part of the World Health Organization. Contrary to the translated name, the IARC does not sponsor or perform cancer research; instead, the organization compiles global publications and evidence for review by panels of scientists. Like the National Academy of Sciences panels, the scientific committees of the IARC are composed of groups of independent scientists, which make decisions and arrive at their findings through the full agreement of all present.

The key findings of IARC committees are contained in periodically updated monographs. Each monograph lays out the available evidence and strength of evidence supporting or refuting links between environmental exposures and cancer. Widely respected, these IARC publications employ a valuable system of ratings that reflect the nature of the evidence and the certainty of the IARC's findings.

- Group 1 agents have been *conclusively* determined to be carcinogenic to humans. Agents in this category include asbestos, benzene, and etopside (a chemotherapy agent), as well as HIV and solar radiation.

- Group 2A agents are considered to be *probably* carcinogenic to humans and include diesel engine exhaust, anabolic steroids, and the most prevalent chemical contaminant in my hometown, PCBs.

- Group 2B agents are considered to be *possibly* carcinogenic to humans and include agents from carbon black to toluene diisocyanates.

- Group 3 agents have been evaluated by the IARC, but the committees lack sufficient quality information to classify them.

- Group 4 agents have been rated as "probably not carcinogenic to humans."[5]

Though science can never "prove" anything with finality, it brings an understanding of possibilities and a degree of certainty based on accumulated evidence. Deciding what evidence is conclusive and choosing what to believe is, in the end, a personal choice. We must decide what to believe given our own experiences and readings of all the evidence.

And we must also learn to read between the lines, because there are times when the relevant research is either left undone or left unpublished. In February 2008, for example, news broke that a well-respected senior administrator and toxicologist at the Centers for Disease Control and Prevention, Christopher De Rosa, was stripped of his supervisory role when he sought to publish a comprehensive review of the effects of toxic chemicals in twenty-six "areas of concern" surrounding the Great Lakes in the United States.

Unauthorized versions of the report were posted on the Internet by the Center for Public Integrity, and De Rosa discussed his work with the media, claiming that the report had been withheld because it was too alarming for the public.[6] He told interviewers for *Living on Earth* on National Public Radio, for example, that the report included evidence of infertility problems and immune deficits and increased breast, colon, and lung cancers in the areas of concern.[7] Under pressure from Congress, the report was later released to the public along with the caveat that it will undergo further review by other agencies and scientists.[8]

As this case demonstrates, the same processes that create knowledge can be organized in such a way that they manufacture controversy and deliver only uncertainty. In a letter to the head of the Centers for Disease Control and Prevention, U.S. Representatives John Dingell and Bart Stupak, Democrats from Michigan, wrote that the handling of the study "raises grave questions about the integrity of scientific research."[9]

In the past, when people told and retold their individual stories of illness, they were delivering narratives that, when knitted together, created a reliable early warning system for others of the dangers present either in nature or in the factory. But today, as we have seen, the link between place and disease can be hard to discover and is stretched out over time and space. The environmental factors that we currently face work with such nuanced complexity in our bodies that it has become almost impossible to tell a simple story with a clear line of causality. Instead, we must tell more complicated stories, with carefully worded conclusions.

Waiting until we have bulletproof lab results or the perfect epidemiological study that will implicate this or that chemical with certainty is a fool's game. We are all exposed to multiple chemicals throughout our lifetimes. Some of the most important exposures come in utero and set off a cascade of genetic changes that cannot be undone and whose effects we are only beginning to understand. Furthermore, each of us has a particular genetic makeup that may make us more or less susceptible to a given chemical exposure in ways not yet fully understood. And, finally, we all carry extensive chemical body burdens. This not only affects the impact of further exposures, but also makes it increasingly challenging for scientists to find a control group of people with no exposure.

In the absence of studies conducted to establish statistical significance, sometimes we must listen to stories and investigate patterns they may hold. For example, it took only six cases of what was then believed to be juvenile rheumatoid arthritis for two mothers in Lyme, Connecticut, working with a map and some stick pins in the 1970s, to discover what we now know as tick-borne Lyme disease. Similarly, eight cases of a rare vaginal cancer were enough to show doctors at a Harvard teaching hospital that a female hormone, diethylstilbestrol (DES), administered during pregnancy, could result many years later in genital cancers in the daughters of the women who took the drug.[10]

Stories matter. In conjunction with other forms of evidence, they can give us the knowledge we need to take informed actions that can help protect future generations. We have waged mammoth and successful public-health battles in this country in the face of complex disease patterns and uncertainty, and we have benefited enormously. We have removed lead from gasoline and paint, helping to safeguard the intelligence of children. We have banned cigarette smoking in airplanes and many public places, and that move alone has helped to lower the chemical byproducts of secondhand smoke found in the blood of bystanders, young and old, nationwide. The banning of PCBs and DDT caused a tremendous drop in the levels of these chemicals in Great Lakes fish, even if those levels remain of considerable concern. The fact that we no longer manufacture goods with asbestos in this country has helped us avoid many thousands of workplace-related illnesses.

These public-health battles have been won by and large based on what I referred to as regulatory proof—the evidential array that regulators need in order to act. This may not be the same quality of "proof" as that needed in a lawsuit, but nevertheless can constitute strong evidence that the risk of harm or further harm is too great to delay action. There is no question in my mind that regulation works, and we need more of it when it comes to the manufacture, use, and disposal of harmful substances.

We could, for example, require that chemicals be tested and approved before they are used widely in consumer goods such as water bottles and baby bottles—instead of waiting until their health effects unfold in future generations. Such policies would be consistent with the kind of environmental leadership the United States was once known for, and it would be consistent with recent regulatory moves in the European Union under its Registration, Evaluation, Authorization, and Restriction of Chemicals (REACH) program.[11]

My town of Waukegan, as dirty as it was and as imperfect as it continues to be, stands out as a constant reminder that we can make progress against the kinds of chemicals that worked their way into the water, into the fabric of the town, into the fish in the lake, and finally and fatally into my sister. Environmentally related cancers and other diseases do not have to be an inevitable outcome of modern life. They are only the likely outcome of the way that we currently produce, purchase, discard, and regulate. We can change those things, if only we care enough to do so.

Epilogue

IF THE CHEMICALS IN Lake Michigan created a massive storm that has buffeted my family for decades, the effects of that storm were equally dramatic in my hometown. Waukegan lost close to 35,000 jobs between the time when the pollution was officially discovered in the early 1970s and the time when the final major polluter on the lakefront went bankrupt in 2001.[1] The closing of the factories sent Waukegan into a deep and sustained economic crisis that ironically coincided with another similarly dramatic economic crisis hundreds of miles away.

For years, poor Mexican *campesinos* had been leaving farmlands to seek work in Mexico City, but a 1995 currency crisis caused a massive devaluation of the peso. As the value of the peso dropped precipitously—by almost 1,000 percent—widespread economic distress led many people to head north in search of work, some making their way to the Chicago area. Waukegan, Ray Bradbury's hometown and mine, continues to be a beacon for immigrants.

"We are the dream that other people dream," wrote Bradbury in "America," a poem published in the *Wall Street Journal* in 2006. "In tides of immigrants that this year flow, we still remain the beckoning hearth they'd know."[2]

Like the Lithuanians, Germans, and Irish immigrants before them, Hispanics streamed into town. Of the nearly 90,000 Waukegan residents counted in the 2000 census, about 39,000 were Hispanic, and many observers believe the actual number is considerably higher. White flight, suburban decay, and Mexican immigration have turned Bradbury's Green Town into what locals now call Bean Town for its many excellent Mexican restaurants. As a result, Waukegan in this new chapter of its history faces a triple challenge. The town must grapple with persistent pollution on its shores, a new immigrant population, and the stigma of its blighted past. In October 2005, *Chicago Magazine* called the town one of the dirtiest in the region, placing a small skull and crossbones beside its name to make the point.[3]

Economic and ethnic tensions in Waukegan have sometimes run high.[4] On one hot July night in 2007, hundreds of the town's Hispanic population rallied in front of city hall to oppose a measure that would give city police officers the ability to start deportation proceedings against undocumented aliens. Carrying signs that read "We Are America," they faced off against a mix of anti-immigration groups and angry locals waving enormous flags and singing "God Bless America."

I watched the confrontation from behind a line of police on the city hall steps, where officers stood silently between the two groups. Some of the police held attack dogs, others were perched high on horseback, while snipers stood alert on rooftops overhead armed with guns and cameras to videotape the unrest. The two groups chanted and harassed each other for over two hours. Even if I couldn't understand their Spanish, I understood the fear and desperation among the Hispanic demonstrators; meanwhile, the hatred coming from the anti-immigration group was palpable.

Midway through the protest, I was approached by a tall, Anglo reporter. She asked what I thought of the demonstration. When I told her I could only understand this angry clash as part of a chain of events that began with the dumping of polluted fluid in the lake decades before, she rolled her eyes and went in search of a better sound bite.

Environmental reporting, urban reporting, all reporting really, is about covering people's hopes and dreams for the future and trying to make sense of the situation they face and the steps they must take to turn their dreams into reality. Casey Bukro covered the Great Lakes and the pollution in Waukegan Harbor for the *Chicago Tribune* from the 1970s until he retired in 2007. "I always thought while covering Waukegan Harbor that I was not just covering technical issues," he told me. "I was covering a dream about the future of Waukegan, and what that community could be once the stigma of a blighted community was lifted. That's what environmental reporting is all about—you have to understand the dream that people have for the place where they live."[5]

The questions for Waukegan are whose dream and, importantly, who pays for the dream. The mayor wants to build luxury condos on the lakefront, but to make those condos a reality he will need to find the money to clean up the polluted areas and also find a way to cope with the waves of newcomers who are currently overwhelming city services.

In 2005, the town hired the architectural firm of Skidmore, Owings and Merrill to prepare a master plan showcasing how the lakefront could be developed. The colorful drawings dot the mayor's office and include luxury shops, condos, and expensive facilities for docking pleasure craft. Some have estimated that the plan would require hundreds of millions of dollars in investment. And that does not include the funds needed to clean up lingering contamination of many lakefront areas.[6] Waukegan is clearly caught between its polluted legacy and its dreams for the future.

"It is difficult to imagine a greater disconnect between the existing environmental constraints to redevelopment and the new lakefront plan," wrote members of a local residents' group. "Some of these proposed residences would not only sit over contaminated soils, but would also lie within close proximity to several pollution-containment cells, including a sealed-off slip that contains PCB-laden sediment dredged from the bottom of the Waukegan harbor."[7]

The juxtaposition of luxury shops and high-end condos next to the Superfund sites seems like something worthy of a Bradbury-type science fiction fantasy. Some thirty years after the vast amounts of PCBs were discovered in Waukegan, the town continues to be an environmental hotspot, with some sediments along the public beach still containing PCBs at a rate of 14,000 parts per million.

The downward spiral that has gripped Waukegan has similarly strangled communities that have major pollution problems all over this country.[8] It happens like this: Large-scale pollution drives down property prices and drives away anyone who can afford to live elsewhere. Depressed property prices attract people with little money and no political clout, and they are seldom in a position to fight effectively against the expansion of pollution-producing facilities and for the necessary cleanups—especially remediation of the magnitude that Waukegan continues to require.

Even the areas that were once treated are still polluted by today's standards. The 1993 Outboard Marine Corporation cleanup brought sediments within the harbor to 50 parts per million—a level that was set by the Toxic Substances Control Act and agreed upon by the U.S. EPA and the company at the time. "Fifty parts per million was a political number," says the EPA's Kevin Adler, who has worked on the site. "That was the number that people could agree on in the 1980s based on the factors in place then—economically and politically—and based on what we knew about PCBs."9

Today, the new standards are much lower, whether those levels relate to fish, to drinking water, or to soil near housing. The standard for soils around high-density housing of the type the Waukegan master plan envisions, for example, is 1 part per million.

The EPA concluded a review of the condition of the harbor and the adjacent Outboard Marine site in September 2007. Mary Gade, an EPA official, called the results "troubling." "Unacceptably high levels of polychlorinated biphenyls still remain in the harbor sediment," she said, "contaminating fish and threatening the health of people and wildlife."10

The EPA, working within the confines of the Great Lakes Legacy Act of 2002, could have provided $24 million for additional cleanup work, but wrangling between city and county officials over how to come up with the necessary $12 million in local matching funds caused the deal to collapse. In the end, local officials let perhaps the town's best chance to clean up its shores slip through their fingers. Without funding from the Great Lakes Legacy Act, and because the parties responsible for the pollution have since gone out of business, cleanup monies will now have to come from the general Superfund. However, monies for the Superfund have historically come from a tax on oil companies, and since 1995 Congress has refused to reinstate the tax—despite the fact that oil companies' profits are skyrocketing. As a result, progress on orphaned sites such as the ones in Waukegan has been perilously slow.

After watching the demonstrators that hot night in July, I drove down to the town beach where I used to play with my sister as a child. The water was clearer and more blue than ever—the result of the zebra mussel, an invasive species that eats almost everything in sight and in the process is killing off native biota and turning the once dark waters a crystal Caribbean blue.

The water was as cold as I remembered, and the wind was sending waves crashing onto the shore. The coal-fired power plant—a fixture on the lakefront for over eighty years and still one of the dirtiest in the nation—continued to belch pollutants into the air. And beneath me a toxic mass of groundwater, a legacy from the town's industrial era, was making its slow but steady way toward the open water.

I sat down and watched two small children kick a soccer ball between them. When my sister handed my infant son back to me as she lay dying, she said to me simply, "He is the future." Her words echoed in my mind as I watched the children play. Those children are the future of Waukegan, I thought, and I mumbled a short prayer for them, a mother's blessing.

As I stood to leave, I grabbed a stone and tossed it into the lake, remembering the afternoons my sister and I had spent doing that very same thing on that same beach so long ago. I thought of all I had been through, all that my sister had gone through, and all that the town had been through. I turned and walked back up the beach to my car—knowing that I would never be able to escape the long reach of that lake.

Acknowledgments

I STARTED THIS BOOK TO fulfill a promise I made to my sister on her deathbed: to investigate what relationship there might be between the pollution in our hometown and her ovarian cancer. In the midst of that research, my own cancer was discovered, and the book about my sister and her illness turned out to be a book about the two of us, Lake Michigan, and the role of toxic chemicals in our illnesses.

During the course of writing this book, I have learned many things, but the one truth I hold dear is this: my sister's death saved me. If she had not had her cancer, I would not have known to look for mine. If she had not made me agree to write this book, my own interest in the subject would have waned and my own health would have been jeopardized; indeed my life might have been cut short. This book, then, represents a promise fulfilled, its reward realized.

It would be a mistake, however, to think that I wrote this book only for my sister. While I set out to tell a very personal story, what I discovered was a universal one. We all carry significant chemical burdens in our bodies today and, as a result, a significant responsibility to try to understand what effect they have on our health and on that of generations to come. This book, then, is for all our children: hers, yours, mine. They are the future.

I would like to thank my agents, Jim Levine and Lindsay Edgecombe of Levine Greenberg. At Island Press, Jonathan Cobb skillfully edited and shepherded this book from its earliest stages. Emily Davis read drafts and offered excellent suggestions. Julie Van Pelt was a fine reader and copyeditor. Chuck Savitt, president of Island Press, was a strong supporter from the beginning and helped to arrange financial backing for the research the book required. I am also grateful to Dr. Lucy R. Waletzky and Catherine Conover for providing additional support.

The advice and encouragement of Madge Kaplan, currently the director of communications for the Institute for Healthcare Improvement and formerly an editor and healthcare correspondent for *Marketplace* and National Public Radio, were invaluable, as was the advice that came from Professor Margaret Quinn at the University of Massachusetts, Lowell. Dr. Kate Adams read and reviewed the manuscript and helped with research as well. Karen Peabody O'Brien of the Center for the Advancement of Green Chemistry was also helpful in shaping early versions of this book. Professor Steve Rosswurm of Lake Forest College helped me understand the history of northern Illinois. Professor Margaret Beattie Bogue from the University of Wisconsin at Madison helped me understand the history of Great Lakes fisheries. Canadian researcher Michael Gilbertson helped me understand the role that toxins play in the health of gulls and other birds of the Great Lakes.

This book took shape over four residencies provided by the Ragdale Foundation in Lake Forest, Illinois. From my base at Ragdale, I was able to tour toxic-waste sites and peruse documents in my hometown of Waukegan. I could not have accomplished this without the help and support of those at Ragdale, including Susan Page Tillett, Sylvia Brown, Melissa Mosher, Jack Danch, and Regin Igloria. I also gratefully acknowledge a stay at the Mesa Writer's Refuge in Point Reyes, California, in 2004 and would like to thank Peter Barnes and the Common Counsel Foundation for arranging it. Alexis Rizzuto and members of the master memoir class at Grub Street in Boston also read portions of the manuscript and offered valuable critiques. Family and friends provided emotional support and patience throughout my extended illness and the long process of writing this book. They include Andrea Sussman and Andrew Troop, Charles Styron and Nancy Frumer-Styron, Sheila and Gary Fireman, Jean Pagani, Ruth Kotlier, and the extended Kotlier clan.

I am deeply indebted to my nephew, who encouraged me to write his mother's story. My son, Jacob, was a constant source of inspiration and energy. Finally, I must thank my husband, Jonathan Kotlier, who supported me both emotionally and financially throughout my illness and the long days, months, and years of writing.

$\mathcal{N}otes$

1. THE USED-CAR SALESMAN'S DAUGHTERS

1. J. P. Zabolski, *The Man from Waukegan* (Lulu.com, 2005), 39. Occasionally, I have turned to historical documents to confirm my childhood memories. This book, for example, paints a vivid description of the lakefront ringed by factories in my hometown.

2. Lee Davis, *Environmental Disasters: A Chronicle of Individual, Industrial and Governmental Carelessness* (New York: Facts on File, 1998), 87.

3. In late 1960s and early 1970s, there was anecdotal evidence of the pollution along the shore and in other parts of town. The first investigations from the Illinois Environmental Protection Agency probably began as early as 1971. However, 1976 is the date most often cited in court cases as the date when the sites were "discovered." This date coincides with some of the earliest regulatory actions concerning toxins in Waukegan by federal authorities.

4. Interview with Margaret Quinn, 2003.

5. See Marla Cone, "Common Chemicals Are Linked to Breast Cancer," *Los Angeles Times*, May 14, 2007, p. A1.

6. Linda Nash, *Inescapable Ecologies: A History of the Environment, Disease and Knowledge* (Berkeley: University of California Press, 2007), 211.

2. GREEN TOWN

1. Illinois Environmental Protection Agency, *Waukegan Remedial Action Plan: Stage I and II Final Report* (Springfield: Illinois Environmental Protection Agency, 1994), 11.

2. See, for example, Louise Osling and Julia Osling, *Historical Highlights of the Waukegan Area* (Waukegan, IL: City of Waukegan, 1976), 27; and William Ashworth, *The Late, Great Lakes* (New York: Knopf, 1986), 175.

3. Ashworth, *The Late, Great Lakes*, 174.

4. Joel Greenberg, *A Natural History of the Great Lakes* (Chicago: University of Chicago Press, 2002), 171.

5. Jeffrey L. Rodengen, *Evinrude-Johnson and the Legend of OMC* (Ft. Lauderdale, FL: Write Stuff Syndicate, 1993).

6. Interview with Professor Steve Rosswurm, Lake Forest College, July 2007.

7. Osling and Osling, *Historical Highlights of the Waukegan Area*, 105.

8. Greenberg, *Natural History of the Great Lakes*, 171.

9. Rachel Carson, *Silent Spring* (Boston: Houghton Mifflin, 1962), 5.

10. League of Women Voters of Waukegan, *Waukegan, Illinois: Its Past, Its Present*, 3rd ed. (Waukegan, IL: League of Women Voters, 1967).

11. Ann L. Greer, *The Mayor's Mandate: Municipal Statecraft and Political Trust* (Rochester, VT: Schenkman Publishing, 1974), 11.

12. Quotations from Sabonjian are from Greer, *Mayor's Mandate*, 45.

13. Greer, *Mayor's Mandate*, 23.

14. Kenan Heise and Edward Baumann, *Chicago Originals* (Chicago: Bonus Books, 1990), 28.

15. "J-M on the Ropes: Asks Chapter 11, Cites Suits," *Waukegan News-Sun*, August 26, 1982, p. 1.

16. Casey Bukro, "Waukegan Hopes Plant Closing Ends PCB Stigma City Seeks New Uses for OMC Facility Area," *Chicago Tribune*, September 27, 1998, p. 1.

17. Robert Cross, "His Honor, the Rock," *Chicago Tribune*, September 26, 1976, p. 19.

18. Ray Bradbury, *Zen in the Art of Writing: Essays on Creativity* (New York: Bantam, 1992), 84.

3. COHO CAPITAL OF THE WORLD

1. See Scott Fields, "Great Lakes: Resources at Risk," *Environmental Health Perspectives* 113, no. 3 (March 2005): A164–173; and John Karl, "Toxic Chemicals Killed All Young Lake Trout in Lake Ontario for 40 Years," *Littoral Drift* (November/December 2003), newsletter of University of Wisconsin Sea Grant Institute, www.seagrant.wisc.edu. Article can be found at: http://www .seagrant.wisc.edu/communications/news/documents/DriftNov Dec 03_000.pdf.

2. Joel Greenberg, *A Natural History of the Chicago Region* (Chicago: University of Chicago Press, 2002), 161.

3. Jerry Dennis, *The Living Great Lakes: Searching for the Heart of the Inland Seas* (New York: St. Martins, 2003), 189.

4. Dennis, *Living Great Lakes*, 189.

5. Dennis, *Living Great Lakes*, 191.

6. Anthony Netboy, *The Salmon: Their Fight for Survival* (Boston: Houghton Mifflin, 1974), 515.

7. Virginia Mullery, *Lake County, Illinois, This Land of Lakes and Rivers: An Illustrated History* (Waukegan, IL: Windsor Publications, 1989; produced in cooperation with the Waukegan/Lake County Chamber of Commerce).

8. Dennis, *Living Great Lakes*, 194.

9. U.S. Environmental Protection Agency, *The Great Lakes: An Environmental Atlas and Resource Book*, 3rd ed., 1995, www.epa. gov/glnpo/atlas.

10. John Rousmaniere, ed., *The Enduring Great Lakes* (New York: W. W. Norton, 1979), 69.

11. William Ashworth, *Great Lakes Journey: A New Look at America's Freshwater Coast* (Detroit: Wayne State University Press, 2000), 52.

12. Different governmental agencies have different tolerance

levels for chemicals in fish. The U.S. Environmental Protection Agency, the U.S. Food and Drug Administration, and many state governments all issue their own guidelines for acceptable limits of chemicals in fish. In addition, these governmental bodies all have the ability to order fish advisories. Moreover, there are different standards for commercial fish and fish caught by recreational fisherman. For one discussion of this issue, please see Environmental Protection Agency, PCB Update on Fish Advisories, September 1999, http://fn.cfs.purdue.edu/fish4health/HealthRisks/PCB.pdf.

13. "Salmon and PCBs," Fox River Watch, www.foxriverwatch.com/salmon_pcb_pcbs.html.

14. Ashworth, *Great Lakes Journey*, 174.

4. THE FALSE CENTER OF THE COLLAGE

1. See William J. Hoskins, *Principles and Practice of Gynecologic Oncology* (Philadelphia: Lippincott, 1995), 31.

2. While I knew of the general concerns about women eating Great Lakes fish at the time of my sister's diagnosis in 1992, the *Epidemiology* study was not published until 2000. See G. M. Buck, J. E. Vena, E. F. Schisterman, J. Dmochowski, P. Mendola, L. E. Sever, E. Fitzgerald, P. Kostyniak, et al., "Prenatal Consumption of Contaminated Sport Fish from Lake Ontario and Predicted Fecundability," *Epidemiology* 11:388–93.

3. According to the *New York Times*, "A study published . . . by Dr. Alice Whittemore at Stanford University had found that women treated with fertility drugs who later went on to have children were three times as likely as their peers to develop ovarian cancer, while those women who did not succeed in getting pregnant were 27 times as likely to develop the disease." See Katherine Bouton, "After the Ball," *New York Times*, April 12, 1998. The original study by Dr. Whittemore is "The Risk of Ovarian Cancer after Treatment for Infertility," *New England Journal of Medicine* 331, no. 12 (1994): 804–6.

4. This article would later become a book. See Liz Tilberis, *No Time to Die* (Boston: Little, Brown, 1998).

5. Lake Michigan Legacy

1. Sheldon Krimsky, *Hormonal Chaos: The Scientific and Social Origins of the Environmental Endocrine Hypothesis* (Baltimore: Johns Hopkins University Press, 2000), 51.

2. P. Grandjean and P. J. Landrigan, "Developmental Neurotoxicity of Industrial Chemicals," *Lancet*, November 2006. See a news report online at *Science Daily*, www.sciencedaily.com/releases /2006/11/061108155004.htm.

3. William Ashworth, *The Late, Great Lakes*, (New York: Knopf, 1986), 176.

4. Outboard Marine Chronology of Events, document created by the Waukegan Historical Society, May 6, 1987.

5. Sandra Steingraber, *Having Faith: An Ecologist's Journey to Motherhood* (Cambridge, MA: Perseus Publishing, 2001), 143.

6. Quoted in Eric Francis, "Conspiracy of Silence: How Three Corporate Giants Covered Their Toxic Trail," *Sierra*, September/ October 2004, www.planetwaves.net/silence2.html.

7. Rachel Carson, *Silent Spring* (Boston: Houghton Mifflin, 1962), 7.

8. *Biphenyls* is the word used to describe the two modified benzene rings; because each benzene ring contains two or more chlorine atoms, biphenyls are called *polychlorinated*. See Ashworth, *Late, Great Lakes*, 177.

9. Roberta C. Barbalace, "The Chemistry of Polychlorinated Biphenyls," EnvironmentalChemistry.com, http://Environmental-Chemistry.com/yogi/chemistry/pcb.html. See also Ashworth, *Late Great Lakes*, 176.

10. Francis, "Conspiracy of Silence."

11. Theodora Colborn, Alex Davidson, Sharon Green, R. A. Hodge, C. Ian Jackson, and Richard A. Liroff, *Great Lakes, Great Legacy* (Washington, DC: Conservation Foundation; Ottawa, ON: Institute for Research on Public Policy, 1990), 138.

12. Colborn, *Great Lakes, Great Legacy*, 138, 139.

13. See G. R. Hartsough, "Great Lakes Fish Now Suspect as Mink Food," *American Fur Breeder* 38 (1965): 24–35.

14. Ashworth, *Late, Great Lakes,* 177.

15. Poul Harremoës, David Gee, Malcolm MacGarvin, Andy Stirling, Jane Keys, Brian Wynne, and Sofia Guedes Vaz, eds., *Late Lessons from Early Warnings: The Precautionary Principle 1896–2000,* Environmental Issue Report no. 22 (Copenhagen: European Environment Agency, 2002), 65, http://reports.eea. europa.eu/environmental_issue_report_2001_22/en/#contents.

16. "Perils of PCBs," *Time* Magazine, May 10, 1976.

17. In the year 1974 alone, Monsanto produced 40 million pounds of PCBs, down from 85 million pounds in 1970. John Harte, Cheryl Holdren, Richard Schneiderand, and Christine Shirley, *Toxics A to Z* (Berkeley: University of California Press, 1991), 387.

18. Interview with Theo Colborn, 2006.

19. Francis, "Conspiracy of Silence." See also "Perils of PCBs," *Time* Magazine, May 10, 1976.

20. "Perils of PCBs," *Time* Magazine, May 10, 1976.

21. Ashworth, *Late, Great Lakes,* 176.

22. Jeffrey L. Rodengen, *Evinrude-Johnson and the Legend of OMC* (Ft. Lauderdale, FL: Write Stuff Syndicate, 1993), 67.

23. Ibid.

24. *The Johnson Mariner,* an Outboard Marine publication published in March 1968, available in the collection of the Waukegan Historical Society.

25. Memo from R. Stenberg to R. M. Atkin, March 2, 1976. Document from *U.S. v. OMC and Monsanto,* U.S. District Court for the Northern District of Illinois, Eastern Division, no. 78 C 1004.

26. *USA v. Outboard Marine Corp. and Monsanto Company,* U.S. Court of Appeals, Seventh Circuit, no. 85-1584, argued December 11, 1985.

27. Memo from Stenberg to Atkin.

28. Deposition of the owner of Larsen Marine. Document from *U.S. v. OMC and Monsanto,* U.S. District Court for the Northern District of Illinois, Eastern Division, no. 78 C 1004.

29. Memo from R. M. Atkin to R. Adams, D. Thaxton. Document from *U.S. v. OMC and Monsanto*, U.S. District Court for the Northern District of Illinois, Eastern Division, no. 78 C 1004.

30. Outboard Marine, Chronology of Events, document from the Waukegan Historical Society.

31. The 240,000 parts per million figure is from *People of the State of Illinois v. OMC*, United States Court of Appeals, Seventh Circuit nos. 79-1341, 79-1725; Ashworth, *Late, Great Lakes*, 179, gives the 500,000 parts per million number.

32. League of Women Voters of Waukegan, *Waukegan, Illinois: Its Past, Its Present*, 3rd ed. (Waukegan, IL: League of Women Voters, 1967), 22.

33. Steve Thorp, Waukegan Harbor Case Study, Great Lakes Dredging Team, Publication of the Great Lakes Commission, www.glc.org/dredging/case/waukegan.html.

34. U.S. Environmental Protection Agency, *The PCB Problem in Waukegan*, January 12, 1981; Illinois Environmental Protection Agency, *Waukegan Remedial Action Plan: Stage I and II Final Report* (Springfield: Illinois Environmental Protection Agency, 1994).

35. John H. Hartig and Michael A. Zarull, *Under RAPs: Toward Grassroots Ecological Democracy in the Great Lakes Basin* (Ann Arbor: University of Michigan Press, 1992), 240.

36. League of Women Voters, *Waukegan, Illinois: Its Past and Present,* 85.

37. Illinois Environmental Protection Agency, *Waukegan Remedial Action Plan*, 59.

38. Ralph Zahorik, "Yeoman Creek: The Flow of Pollution Continues," *Waukegan News-Sun*, June 7, 1972.

39. Ann L. Greer, *The Mayor's Mandate: Municipal Statecraft and Political Trust* (Rochester, VT: Schenkman Publishing, 1974), 122.

40. ATSDR, "Public Health Assessment, Yeoman Creek," September 30, 1997, p. 2. A report prepared by the Agency for Toxic Substances and Disease Registry in conjunction with the Illinois Department of Public Health.

41. Interview with David Carpenter, fall 2006.

42. Memo from R. M. Atkin to R. Stenberg, March 5, 1976; Document from *U.S. v. OMC and Monsanto*, U.S. District Court for the Northern District of Illinois, Eastern Division, no. 78 C 1004.

43. Deposition of William Schwartz, formerly of Lester Engineering. Lester Engineering sold the die-casting machines to Outboard Marine. Document from *U.S. v. OMC and Monsanto*, U.S. District Court for the Northern District of Illinois, Eastern Division, no. 78 C 1004.

44. Craig E. Colten and Peter N. Skinner, *The Road to Love Canal* (Austin: University of Texas Press, 1995), preface.

45. Quoted in Kenneth A. Gould, Allan Schnaiberg, and Adam S. Weinberg, *Local Environmental Struggles: Citizen Activism in the Treadmill of Production* (New York: Cambridge University Press, 1996), 102.

46. Hartig and Zarull, *Under RAPs*, 6.

47. Colborn, *Great Lakes, Great Legacy*, xxvi.

48. LeAnn Spencer, "Waukegan Clean Up an EPA Milestone," *Chicago Tribune*, August 4, 1993, p. 1.

49. Robert Proctor, *Cancer Wars: How Politics Shapes What We Know and Don't Know about Cancer* (New York: Basic Books, 1995), 78.

50. Proctor, *Cancer Wars*, 82.

51. Quoted in Proctor, *Cancer Wars*, 80.

52. Spencer, "Waukegan Clean Up an EPA Milestone."

53. Dan Moran, "Going, Going, Soon to Be Gone," *Waukegan News-Sun*, August 31, 2006.

54. Interview with Evan Craig, January 2007.

55. John Lucadamo, "EPA Pushes Waukegan Pond Clean-Up," *Chicago Tribune*, September 21, 1990. In 1990, an emergency cleanup was undertaken to prevent more birds from slowly sinking and drowning in the toxic muck.

56. Interview with an Illinois EPA official, 2007.

6. A Marked Woman

1. For a complete history of the emergence of the endocrine disruptor theory, see Sheldon Krimsky, *Hormonal Chaos: The Scientific and Social Origins of the Environmental Endocrine Hypothesis* (Baltimore, Johns Hopkins University Press, 2000).

2. Interview with Theo Colborn, 2006.

3. Tom Spears, "Great Lakes Toxins Cause Human Infertility," *Ottawa Citizen*, September 23, 1999, http://boating.ncf.ca/newsgl .html.

4. Author's correspondence with her doctors, October 25, 2002.

5. Ibid.

7. Miasma

1. Linda Nash, *Inescapable Ecologies: A History of the Environment, Disease and Knowledge* (Berkeley: University of California Press, 2007). Many of the ideas in this chapter are drawn from this amazing piece of scholarly work.

2. Nash discusses this phenomenon on p. 210 of *Inescapable Ecologies*.

3. Interview with Mayor Richard Hyde, Waukegan, Illinois, January 2007.

4. Sandra Steingraber, *Living Downstream: An Ecologist Looks at Cancer and the Environment* (New York: Addison-Wesley, 1997), 43.

5. Barry Johnson, Heraline Hicks, Annette Ashizawa, Christopher De Rosa, Vincent Cogliano, and Milton Clark, *Public Health Implications of Exposure to Polychlorinated Biphenyls*, Agency for Toxic Substances and Disease Registry, www.atsdr.cdc.gov/ DT/pcb007.html.

6. Quoted in Amy Marcus, "A Cry in the Dark: When a Rare Cancer Strikes, Patient Has Few Places to Turn," *Wall Street Journal*, March 20, 2006, p. R9. Judah Folkman died in 2008.

8. Hitchhiking Hormones

1. Quoted in John Mann, *Life Saving Drugs: The Elusive Magic Bullet* (London: Royal Society of Chemistry, 2004), 141.

2. Robert Proctor, *Cancer Wars: How Politics Shapes What We Know and Don't Know about Cancer* (New York: Basic Books, 1995), 22.

3. James S. Olson, *Bathsheba's Breast: Women, Cancer and History* (Baltimore: Johns Hopkins University Press, 2002), 22.

4. Proctor, *Cancer Wars*, 22.

5. Mann, *Life Saving Drugs*, 142.

6. W. H. Auden, *The Collected Poems: Auden* (New York: Vintage, 1991), 158.

7. Ethel Sloan, *The Biology of Women* (New York: Thomson Delmar Learning; 4th ed., 2001), 50.

8. Natalie Angier, *Woman: An Intimate Geography* (New York: Anchor, 2000), 176.

9. N. Seppa, "Ovulation Linked to Ovarian Cancer," *Science News* 152, no. 1 (July 5, 1997): 7.

10. Susan Love, *Dr. Susan Love's Menopause and Hormone Book: Making Informed Choices* (New York: Three Rivers Press, 1997), 203.

11. Richard W. Clapp, Genevieve K. Howe, and Molly M. Jacobs, *Environmental and Occupational Causes of Cancer: A Review of Recent Scientific Literature* (Lowell: Lowell Center for Sustainable Production, University of Massachusetts, Lowell, 2005). Also available at www.healthandenvironment.org/wg_cancer_news/216. "Although numerous studies have linked perineal use of talc powder with ovarian cancer, some studies have found conflicting results. Based on a meta-analysis of exposure to talc powder comprising 16 studies, researchers found a statistically significant increased risk of ovarian cancer associated with talc exposure, although the evidence was limited by the lack of a clear dose-response relationship" (19).

12. Bill Sells, "What Asbestos Taught Me about Managing Risk," *Harvard Business Review*, March 1, 1994, p. 6.

13. Bernard Harlow, "A Review of Perineal Talc Exposure and Risk of Ovarian Cancer," *Regulatory Toxicology and Pharmacology* 21 (1995): 254–60.

14. See Theo Colborn, Dianne Dumanoski, and John Peterson Myers, *Our Stolen Future* (New York: Plume, 1997).

15. "The incidence of endometriosis seems to have increased in the past 20–50 years and the age of onset seems to have lowered," says Linda Birnbaum, director of the U.S. EPA's Experimental Toxicology Division. Interview with Linda Birnbaum, U.S. EPA toxicologist, December 7, 2006.

16. H. Stefansson, R. T. Geirsson, V. Steinthorsdottir, H. Jonsson, A. Manolescu, A. Kong, G. Ingadottir, J. Gulcher, and K. Stefansson, "Genetic Factors Contribute to the Risk of Developing Endometriosis," *Human Reproduction* 17, no. 3 (March 2002): 555–59.

17. See Amy Davis and Mirka Jones, *Final Diagnosis—Clear Cell Carcinoma of the Ovary.* Case Study of the University of Pittsburgh Medical Center, http://path.upmc.edu/cases/case343/dx.html.

18. Interview with Birnbaum, December 7, 2006.

19. Sherry Rier, W. E. Turner, D. C. Martin, R. Morris, G. W. Lucier, and G. C. Clark. "Serum Levels of TCDD and Dioxin-like Chemicals in Rhesus Monkeys Chronically Exposed to Dioxin: Correlation of Increased Serum PCB Levels with Endometriosis," *Toxicological Sciences* 59 (2001): 147–59 . See also an interview with Linda Birnbaum in *Environmental Review Newsletter* 1, no. 8 (August 1994), www.environmentalreview.org/archives/vol01/birn baum.html.

20. The two studies are discussed in Carol Potera, "Endometriosis and PCB Exposure," *Environmental Health Perspectives* 114, no. 7 (July 2006): A404.

21. Susan J. Elliot, John Eyles, and Patrick Deluca, "Mapping Health in the Great Lakes Area of Concern," *Environmental Health Perspectives* 109 (2001): 817.

22. Centers for Disease Control and Prevention, *Third National Report on Human Exposures to Environmental Chemicals*, NCEH Publication no. 05-0570 (Atlanta: National Center for Environmental Health, 2005), 145, www.cdc.gov/exposurereport/pdf/third report.pdf.

23. Colborn, Dumanoski, and Myers, *Our Stolen Future*, 203.

9. ME TOO

1. Arthur Frank, *The Wounded Storyteller: Body, Illness, and Ethics* (Chicago: University of Chicago Press, 1995), 10.

2. In the days before digital mammograms, radiologists read the screens immediately after they were taken and diagnoses were given that day. More often, today, a letter arrives in the mail a week or two after the screening takes place.

3. Sherwin Nuland, *Wisdom of the Body* (New York: Knopf, 1997), 55.

4. Author's correspondence with her doctors, April 2003.

5. Frank, *Wounded Storyteller*, 158.

6. Will Dunham, "Stem Cell Find Could Advance Pancreatic Cancer Treatment," *Boston Globe*, February 2, 2007, p. A16.

7. L. D. Thompson, R. C. Becker, R. M. Przygodzki, C. F. Adair, and C. S. Heffess, "Mucinous Cystic Neoplasm (Mucinous Cystadenocarcinoma of Low-Grade Malignant Potential) of the Pancreas: A Clinicopathologic Study of 130 Cases," *American Journal of Surgical Pathology* 23, no. 1 (January 1999): 1–16.

8. Andrew Warshaw, William Brugge, Kent Lewondrowski, and Mark Puttman, "Case 35-2003—A 75-year-old Man with a Cystic Lesion of the Pancreas," *New England Journal of Medicine,* Volume 349, no. 20 (November 13, 2003): 1954–61. Although there are few large-scale clinical studies of my disease, *New England Journal of Medicine* recently published a case study of a seventy-five-year-old man with a pancreatic cystic lesion similar to mine. As part of that article, doctors from Massachusetts General Hospital reported their experience with eighty patients diagnosed with mucinous neoplasms treated at their facility. Within that group, there was only one death of a patient in which the disease had not spread. A similar study published in *Gastroenterology* in 2002 reported no deaths of patients where the disease remained isolated (see Hara Yamaguchi and T. Ishihara, "Diagnosis and Patient

Management of Mucinous Tumor of the Pancreas," *Gastroenterology* 122 [2002]: 34–43).

9. This study is discussed in Atul Gawande, *Complications* (New York: Picador, 2003), 220.

10. J. P. Neoptolemos, J. A. Dunn, D. D. Stocken, J. Almond, K. Link, H. Beger, C. Bassi, M. Falconi, P. Pederzoli, C. Dervenis, et al. "Adjuvant Chemoradiotherapy and Chemotherapy in Resectable Pancreatic Cancer: A Randomised Controlled Trial." *Lancet* 358 (2001): 1576–85.

11. Nuland, *Wisdom of the Body,* 62.

12. G. B. Jones, "From Mustard Gas to Medicine: The History of Chemotherapy," *Chemical Heritage* 15, no. 2 (Spring 1998): 8–9, 40–42.

13. Ibid. A group of researchers from the University of Pennsylvania conducted autopsies on seventy-five men who died from mustard gas poisoning during World War I. The U.S. Chemical Warfare Service confirmed its own studies by dosing rabbits with the gas.

14. John Mann, *Life Saving Drugs: The Elusive Magic Bullet* (London: Royal Society of Chemistry, 2004), 159.

15. Ibid.

16. Edmund Russell, *War and Nature: Fighting Humans and Insects with Chemicals from World War 1 to Silent Spring* (Cambridge: Cambridge University Press, 2001), 137.

17. Jennifer Lee, "E.P.A. Relaxes Restrictions on Sale of Contaminated Land," *New York Times,* September 3, 2003.

18. Cathy Newman, "Twelve Toxic Tales," *National Geographic,* May 2005, p. 9.

10. DESTINY

1. Arthur Frank, *The Wounded Storyteller: Body, Illness, and Ethics* (Chicago: University of Chicago Press, 1995), 135–37.

2. Alice Munro, *The Lives of Girls and Women* (New York: Vintage, 2001), 50.

3. Peter Waldman, "Common Industrial Chemicals in Tiny Doses Raise Health Issue," *Wall Street Journal*, July 25, 2005, p. A1.

4. Kirsten Moysich, "Research Commentary: Thoughts on Recent Finds Regarding Organochlorines and Breast Cancer Risk," *The Ribbon* 6, no. 3 (Fall 2001), http://envirocancer.cornell.edu/Newsletter/articles/v6rc.organochlorine.cfm.

5. Robert Proctor, *Cancer Wars: How Politics Shapes What We Know and Don't Know about Cancer* (New York: Basic Books, 1995), 70.

6. See Wayt Gibbs, "Untangling the Roots of Cancer," *Scientific American*, July 2003.

7. Robert Pool, *Environmental Contamination, Biotechnology and the Law: The Impact of Emerging Genomic Information. Summary of a Forum Held at the National Academy of Sciences, August 16, 2000* (Washington, DC: National Academies Press, 2004), 4, http://books.nap.edu/catalog/10104.html.

8. David Biello, "Bringing Cancer to the Dinner Table: Breast Cancer Cells Grow Under Influence of Fish Flesh," *Scientific American*, April 17, 2007. http://www.sciam.com/article.cfm?id=bringing-cancer-to-dinner-table-breast-cancer-cells-grow-under-influence-fish-flesh.

9. Quoted in Pool, *Environmental Contamination, Biotechnology and the Law*, 14.

10. James Olson, *Bathsheba's Breast: Women, Cancer and History* (Baltimore: Johns Hopkins University Press, 2002), 238.

11. Hu Yan, "Number of Cancer Cases Rises Rapidly," *China Daily*, September 20, 2006, www.chinadaily.com.cn/china/2006-09/20/content_692644.htm.

12. Raja Mishra, "New Funding Spurs the Battle Against Pancreatic Cancer," *Boston Globe*, May 23, 2003.

13. Jane Hoppin, P. E. Tolbert, E. A. Holly, J. W. Brock, S. A. Korrick, L. M. Altshul, R. H. Zhang, P. M. Bracci, V. W. Burse, and L. L. Needham, "Pancreatic Cancer and Serum Organochlorine Levels," *Cancer Epidemiology Biomarkers* 9 (2000): 199–205.

14. L. D. Thompson, R. C. Becker, R. M. Przygodzki, C. F.

Adair, and C. S. Heffess, "Mucinous Cystic Neoplasm (Mucinous Cystadenocarcinoma of Low-Grade Malignant Potential) of the Pancreas: A Clinicopathologic Study of 130 Cases" *American Journal of Surgical Pathology* 23, no. 1 (January 1999): 1–16.

15. Ibid.; and R. R. Weihing, I. P. Shintaku, S. A. Geller, and L. M. Petrovic, "Hepatobiliary and Pancreatic Mucinous Cystadenocarcinomas with Mesenchymal Stroma: Analysis of Estrogen Receptors/Progesterone Receptors and Expression of Tumor-Associated Antigens," *Modern Pathology* 10, no. 4 (April 1997): 372–79.

11. WHY ASK WHY?

1. Deborah Mead, "Throwing a Lifeline: Two Friends Deal with a Cancer Diagnosis by Creating Their Own Affirming Ritual," *Boston Globe*, February 8, 2007.

2. *Promise and Progress*, Winter 2006, p. 12, the magazine of the Sidney Kimmel Comprehensive Cancer Center at Johns Hopkins.

3. Robert Proctor, *Cancer Wars: How Politics Shapes What We Know and Don't Know about Cancer* (New York: Basic Books, 1995), 8.

4. Susan Sontag, *Illness as Metaphor* (New York: Picador, 1977), 35.

5. See this animation at http://www.randomhouse.com/knopf/cancervixen/.

6. Arthur Frank, *At the Will of the Body* (Boston: Houghton Mifflin, 1991), 113.

7. Theo Colborn, Dianne Dumanoski, and John Peterson Myers, *Our Stolen Future* (New York: Plume, 1997), 9. This fact is from Denmark, although rates of testicular cancer are thought to have jumped across the board.

8. Arthur Frank, *The Wounded Storyteller: Body, Illness, and Ethics* (Chicago: University of Chicago Press, 1995), 137, 143.

9. Martha Freeman, ed., *Always, Rachel: The Letters of Rachel Carson and Dorothy Freeman* (Boston: Beacon Press, 1996), 401.

10. Ibid.

11. Ibid., 408. The letter is dated June 27, 1962.

12. PROOF

1. See Polly J. Hoppin and Richard Clapp, "Science and Regulation: Current Impasse and Future Solutions," *American Journal of Public Health* 95, S1 (July 2005): S8–S12.

2. For an excellent synopsis and discussion of this case and its implications for public health proceedings in the courts, please see Lawrence Gostin, *Public Health Law and Ethics: A Reader* (Berkeley: University of California Press, 2002), chapter 9, 1–13, http://www.publichealthlaw.net/Reader/docs/GE_Joiner.pdf.

3. *General Electric Company v. Robert K. Joiner*, U.S. Supreme Court, December 15, 1997, 522 U.S. 136 (1997). Chief Justice Rehnquist delivered the opinion of the Court.

4. Sheila Jasanoff, *Science at the Bar* (Cambridge, MA: Harvard University Press, 1997), 59.

5. International Agency for Research on Cancer, IARC Monographs on the Evaluation of Carcinogenic Risks to Humans, Classification of Agents, http://monographs.iarc.fr/ENG/Classification/index.php. IARC ratings have been known to change during successive revisions of monographs. For example, in 1978 the IARC placed PCBs in Group 2B: possible human carcinogen. Additional evidence reviewed in 1987 resulted in a reclassification of PCBs as Group 2A: probable human carcinogen.

6. Sheila Kaplan, "Great Lakes Danger Zones?" *Center for Public Integrity*, February 19, 2008, www.publicintegrity.org/report.aspx?aid=963.

7. "Toxic Info Withheld," *Living on Earth*, February 15, 2008, www.loe.org/shows/segments.htm?programID=08-P13-00007&segmentID=2.

8. Mike Stobbe, "Under Pressure CDC Releases Great Lakes Pollution Report Citing Health Problems," March 12, 2008, Associated Press report can be found at http://climate.weather.com/articles/cdc031308.html.

9. Ibid.

10. Paul Stolley and Tamar Lasky, *Investigating Disease Patterns: The Science of Epidemiology* (New York: Scientific American Library, 1995), 211 (Lyme disease), 146–47 (DES).

11. Mark Schapiro, *Exposed: The Toxic Chemistry of Everyday Products and What's at Stake for American Power* (White River Junction, VT: Chelsea Green Publishing, 2007), 137.

EPILOGUE

1. Dennis Cauchon, "Great Lakes See a Future Beyond Industry," *USA Today*, December 3, 2007.

2. Ray Bradbury, "America," *Wall Street Journal*, May 17, 2006.

3. Cassie Walker, "How Healthy Is Your Town," *Chicago Magazine*, October 2005, p. 89.

4. See the town forums at the website for the *Taskforce on Waukegan Neighborhoods*, www.waukegan.org.

5. Interview with Casey Bukro, March 2007.

6. See the Waukegan master plan on the Skidmore, Owings and Merrill website, www.som.com/content.cfm/waukegan_lakefront _downtown_master_plan.

7. Taskforce on Waukegan Neighborhoods, "T.O.W.N. Lakefront Redevelopment Report," August 10, 2003, p. 3, www. waukegan.org.

8. More than half of all people living within two miles of a hazardous-waste site are minorities. See Robert D. Bullard, *Toxic Wastes and Race at Twenty 1987–2007: Grassroots Struggles to Dismantle Environmental Racism in the United States*, report prepared for the United Church of Christ Justice and Witness Ministries, www.ejrc.cau.edu/TWARTFinal.htm.

9. Interview with Kevin Adler, January 2007.

10. Mary Gade, letter to the *Waukegan News-Sun*, October 30, 2007.

Selected Bibliography

Angier, Natalie. *Woman: An Intimate Geography*. New York: Anchor, 2000.

Arnold, D. L., E. A. Nera, R. Stapley, G. Tolnai, P. Claman, S. Hayward, H. Tryphonas, and F. Bryce, "Prevalence of Endometriosis in Rhesus (*Macaca mulatta*) Monkeys Ingesting PCB (Aroclor 1254): Review and Evaluation." *Fundamental and Applied Toxicology* 31 (May 1996): 42–55.

Ashworth, William. *Great Lakes Journey: A New Look at America's Freshwater Coast*. Detroit: Wayne State University Press, 2000.

———. *The Late, Great Lakes*. New York: Knopf, 1986.

Auden, W. H. *The Collected Poems: Auden*. New York: Vintage, 1991.

Ballweg, Mary Lou. *Endometriosis*. Chicago: Contemporary Books, 2003.

Bogue, Margaret Beattie. *Fishing the Great Lakes: An Environmental History, 1783–1933*. Madison: University of Wisconsin Press, 2000.

Bradbury, Ray. *Zen in the Art of Writing: Essays on Creativity*. New York: Bantam, 1992.

Brodeur, Paul. *Outrageous Misconduct: The Asbestos Industry on Trial*. New York: Pantheon, 1985.

Bullard, Robert D. *Dumping in Dixie: Race, Class and Environmental Quality*. Boulder, CO: Westview, 2000.

———. *Toxic Wastes and Race at Twenty 1987–2007: Grassroots Struggles to Dismantle Environmental Racism in the United States*, report prepared for the United Church of Christ Justice and Witness Ministries. www.ejrc.cau.edu/TWARTFinal.htm.

Carson, Rachel. *Silent Spring*. Boston: Houghton Mifflin, 1962.

Colborn, Theodora, et al. *Great Lakes, Great Legacy*. Washington, DC: Conservation Foundation; Ottawa, ON: Institute for Research on Public Policy, 1990.

Colborn, Theodora, Dianne Dumanoski, and John Peterson Myers. *Our Stolen Future*. New York: Plume, 1997.

Colten, Craig E., and Peter N. Skinner. *The Road to Love Canal: Managing Industrial Waste Before EPA*. Austin: University of Texas Press, 1995.

Cone, Marla. *Silent Snow: The Slow Poisoning of the Arctic*. New York: Grove, 2005.

Cook, P. M., J. A. Robbins, D. D. Endicott, K. B. Lodge, P. D. Guiney, M. K. Walker, E. W. Zabel, and R. E. Peterson. "Effects of Aryl Hydrocarbon Receptor-Mediated Early Life Stage Toxicity on Lake Trout Populations in Lake Ontario during the Twentieth Century." *Environmental Science and Technology* 37 (September 2003): 3864–77.

Cronon, William. *Nature's Metropolis: Chicago and the Great West*. New York: W. W. Norton, 1992.

Davis, Devra. *The Secret History of the War on Cancer*. New York: Perseus, 2007.

———. *When Smoke Ran Like Water: Tales of Environmental Deception and the Battle Against Pollution*. New York: Basic Books, 2000.

Davis, Lee. *Environmental Disasters: A Chronicle of Individual, Industrial and Governmental Carelessness*. Washington, DC: Facts on File, 1988.

Dempsey, Dave. *On the Brink: The Great Lakes in the 21st Century*. East Lansing: Michigan State University Press, 2004.

Dennis, Jerry. *The Living Great Lakes: Searching for the Heart of the Inland Seas*. New York: St. Martin's, 2003.

Dorsey, Curtis L. "Black Migration to Waukegan." Excerpted in *Historical Highlights of the Waukegan Area*. An official publication of the City of Waukegan, 1976.

Durnil, Gordon K. *The Making of a Conservative Environmentalist*. Bloomington: Indiana University Press, 1995.

Egan, Dan. "Paradise in Peril: Lake Michigan Is Showing Signs of Vulnerability—or Even Ecological Breakdown." *Milwaukee Journal Sentinel*, December 11, 2004. www.jsonline.com/index/index.aspx?id=12.

———. "Ships from Overseas Bring Unwelcome Sea Voyagers." *Milwaukee Journal Sentinel*, December 25, 2004. www.jsonline.com/index/index.aspx?id=12.

Eisen, Andy. "Mexican Migration: Chicago's Transnational Suburbs." Senior thesis, Lake Forest College, Lake Forest, IL, 2005.

Faigman, David L. *Legal Alchemy: The Use and Misuse of Science in the Law*. New York: Freeman and Company, 1999.

Fields, Scott. "Great Lakes: Resource at Risk." *Environmental Health Perspectives* 113, no. 3 (March 2005): A164–73.

Francis, Eric. "Conspiracy of Silence: How Three Corporate Giants Covered Their Toxic Trail." *Sierra*, September/October 2004. www.planetwaves.net/silence2.html.

Frank, Arthur. *The Wounded Storyteller: Body, Illness, and Ethics*. Chicago: University of Chicago Press, 1995.

Forrestal, Dan. J. *Faith, Hope and $5,000: The Story of Monsanto*. New York: Simon and Schuster, 1977.

Gibbs, Wayt. "Untangling the Roots of Cancer." *Scientific American*, June 2003.

Golan, Tad. *Laws of Men and Laws of Nature*. Cambridge, MA: Harvard University Press, 2004.

Gould, Kenneth A., Allan Schnaiberg, and Adam S. Weinberg. *Local Environmental Struggles: Citizen Activism in the Treadmill of Production*. New York: Cambridge University Press, 1996.

Greenberg, Joel. *A Natural History of the Chicago Region*. Chicago: University of Chicago Press, 2002.

Greer, Ann L. *The Mayor's Mandate: Municipal Statecraft and Political Trust*. Rochester, VT: Schenkman Publishing, 1974.

Griffiths, Miller. *An Introduction to Genetic Analysis*. New York: Freeman, 2000.

Guarch, Rosa, Ana Puras, Rafael Ceres, M. Alejandra Isaac, and Francisco F. Nogales. "Ovarian Endometriosis and Clear Cell Carcinoma, Leiomyomatosis Peritonealis Disseminata, and Endometrial Adenocarcinoma: An Unusual, Pathogenetically Related Association," *International Journal of Gynecological Pathology* 20, no. 3 (July 2001): 267–70.

Hansen, M. J., and M. E. Holey. "Ecological Factors Affecting the Sustainability of Chinook and Coho Salmon Populations in the Great Lakes, Especially Lake Michigan." In *Sustaining North American Salmon: Perspectives across Regions and Disciplines*, ed. K. D. Lynch, M. L. Jones, and W. W. Taylor. Bethesda, MD: American Fisheries Society, 2002.

Harremoës, Poul, David Gee, Malcolm MacGarvin, Andy Stirling, Jane Keys, Brian Wynne, and Sofia Guedes Vaz, eds. *Late Lessons from Early Warnings: The Precautionary Principle 1896–2000*. Environmental Issue Report no 22. Copenhagen: European Environment Agency, 2002. http://reports.eea. europa.eu/environmental_issue_report_2001_22/en/#contents.

Harte, John, Cherly Holdren, Richard Schneider, and Christine Shirley. *Toxics A to Z: A Guide to Everyday Pollution Hazards*. Berkeley: University of California Press, 1991.

Hartig, John H., and Michael A. Zarull. *Under RAPs: Toward Grassroots Ecological Democracy in the Great Lakes Basin*. Ann Arbor: University of Michigan Press, 1992.

Heise, Kenan, and Edward Baumann. *Chicago Originals*. Chicago: Bonus Books, 1990.

Hoppin, Polly J., and Richard Clapp. "Science and Regulation: Current Impasse and Future Solutions." *American Journal of Public Health* 95, S1 (2005): S8–S12.

Hoskins, William J. *Principles and Practice of Gynecologic Oncology*. Philadelphia: Lippincott, 1995.

Illinois Environmental Protection Agency. *Waukegan Remedial Action Plan: Stage I and II Final Report*. Springfield: Illinois Environmental Protection Agency, 1994.

Jasanoff, Sheila. *Science at the Bar: Law, Science, and Technology in America.* Cambridge, MA: Harvard University Press 1995.

Jones, G. B. "From Mustard Gas to Medicine: The History of Chemotherapy." *Chemical Heritage*15, no. 2 (Spring 1998): 8–9, 40–42.

Judson, Horace Freeland. *The Great Betrayal: Fraud in Science.* New York: Harcourt, 2004.

Just, Ward. *A Family Trust.* New York: Public Affairs, 1978.

Kaplan, Sheila. "Great Lakes Danger Zones?" *Center for Public Integrity*, February 19, 2008. www.publicintegrity.org/report.aspx?aid=963.

Kleinman, Arthur. *The Illness Narratives: Suffering, Healing and the Human Condition.* New York: Basic Books, 1989.

Krimsky, Sheldon. *Hormonal Chaos: The Scientific and Social Origins of the Environmental Endocrine Hypothesis.* Baltimore: Johns Hopkins University Press, 2000.

Kroll, Steve. *Illness and the Environment: A Reader in Contested Medicine.* New York: New York University Press, 2000.

League of Women Voters of Waukegan. *Waukegan, Illinois: Its Past, Its Present.* 3rd ed. Waukegan, IL: League of Women Voters, 1967.

Leopold, Aldo. *A Sand County Almanac and Sketches Here and There.* New York: Oxford University Press, 1949.

Link, Ed. *A Chronology of Waukegan from 1674 to 1997.* Waukegan: Waukegan Historical Society, 1997.

Love, Susan. *Dr. Susan Love's Menopause and Hormone Book: Making Informed Choices.* New York: Three Rivers Press, 1997.

Mann, John. *Life Saving Drugs: The Elusive Magic Bullet.* London: Royal Society of Chemistry, 2004.

Markowitz, Gerald, and David Rosner. *Deceit and Denial: The Deadly Politics of Industrial Pollution.* Berkeley: University of California Press, 2002.

Moyers, Bill. "A Question for Journalists: How Do We Cover Penguins and the Politics of Denial?" Speech before the Society of Environmental Journalists, Austin, TX, October 1, 2005.

Mullery, Virginia. *Lake County, Illinois: This Land of Lakes and Rivers: An Illustrated History.* Waukegan, IL: Windsor Publications, 1989. Produced in cooperation with the Waukegan/Lake County Chamber of Commerce.

Munro, Alice. *The Lives of Girls and Women.* New York: Vintage, 2001.

Nash, Linda. *Inescapable Ecologies: A History of the Environment, Disease and Knowledge.* Berkeley: University of California Press, 2007.

Neoptolemos, J. P., J. A. Dunn, D. D. Stocken, J. Almond, K. Link, H. Beger, C. Bassi, M. Falconi, P. Pederzoli, C. Dervenis, et al. "Adjuvant Chemoradiotherapy and Chemotherapy in Resectable PancreaticCancer: A Randomised Controlled Trial." *Lancet* 358 (2001): 1576–85.

Nestle, Marion. *What to Eat.* New York: North Point Press, 2006.

Netboy, Anthony. *The Salmon: Their Fight for Survival.* Boston: Houghton Mifflin, 1974.

Nuland, Sherwin. *How We Die: Reflections on Life's Final Chapters.* New York: Vintage, 1995.

———. *Wisdom of the Body.* New York: Knopf, 1997.

Olson, James S. *Bathsheba's Breast: Women, Cancer and History.* Baltimore: Johns Hopkins University Press, 2002.

Osling, Louise, and Julia Osling. *Historical Highlights of the Waukegan Area.* Waukegan, IL: City of Waukegan, 1976.

Pool, Robert. *Environmental Contamination, Biotechnology and the Law: The Impact of Emerging Genomic Information; Summary of a Forum Held at the National Academy of Sciences, August 16, 2000.* Washington, DC: National Academies Press, 2004. http://books.nap.edu/catalog/10104.html.

Proctor, Robert. *Cancer Wars: How Politics Shapes What We Know and Don't Know about Cancer.* New York: Basic Books, 1995.

Ridley, Matt. *Genome: The Autobiography of a Species in 23 Chapters.* New York: HarperCollins, 2000.

Rodengen, Jeffrey L. *Evinrude-Johnson and the Legend of OMC.* Ft. Lauderdale, FL: Write Stuff Syndicate, 1993.

Rousmaniere, John, ed. *The Enduring Great Lakes*. New York: W. W. Norton, 1979.

Russell, Edmund. *War and Nature: Fighting Humans and Insects with Chemicals from World War 1 to Silent Spring*. Cambridge: Cambridge University Press, 2001.

Schapiro, Mark. *Exposed: The Toxic Chemistry of Everyday Products and What's at Stake for American Power*. White River Junction, VT: Chelsea Green, 2007.

Sloane, Ethel. *Biology of Women*. 4th ed. New York: Thomson Delmar Learning, 2001.

Sontag, Susan. *Illness as Metaphor and AIDS and Its Metaphors*. New York: Picador, 1977.

Stefansson, H., R. T. Geirsson, V. Steinthorsdottir, H. Jonsson, A. Manolescu, A. Kong, G. Ingadottir, J. Gulcher, and K. Stefansson. "Genetic Factors Contribute to the Risk of Developing Endometriosis," *Human Reproduction* 17, no. 3 (March 2002): 555–59.

Steingraber, Sandra. *Having Faith: An Ecologist's Journey to Motherhood*. Cambridge, MA: Perseus, 2001.

———. *Living Downstream: An Ecologist Looks at Cancer and the Environment*. New York: Addison-Wesley, 1997.

Stolley, Paul D., and Tamar Lasky. *Investigating Disease Patterns: The Science of Epidemiology*. New York: Scientific American Library, 1995.

Thompson, L. D., R. C. Becker, R. M. Przygodzki, C. F. Adair, and C. S. Heffess. "Mucinous Cystic Neoplasm (Mucinous Cystadenocarcinoma of Low-Grade Malignant Potential) of the Pancreas: A Clinicopathologic Study of 130 Cases." *American Journal of Surgical Pathology* 23, no. 1 (January 1999): 1–16.

U.S. Environmental Protection Agency. *The Great Lakes: An Environmental Atlas and Resource Book*. 3rd ed. 1995. www.epa. gov/glnpo/atlas.

Weinberg, Robert. *One Renegade Cell*. New York: Basic Books, 1998.

Weller, Sam. *The Bradbury Chronicles: The Life of Ray Bradbury;*

Predicting the Past, Remembering the Future. New York: William Morrow, 2005.

Wexler, Alice. *Mapping Fate: A Memoir of Family, Risk, and Genetic Research*. New York: Times Books/Random House, 1995.

Wilson, Edward O. *The Future of Life*. New York: Vintage Books, 1971.

Zabolski, J. P. *The Man from Waukegan*. 2005. Lulu.com.

Index

About Island Press

Since 1984, the nonprofit Island Press has been stimulating, shaping, and communicating the ideas that are essential for solving environmental problems worldwide. With more than 800 titles in print and some 40 new releases each year, we are the nation's leading publisher on environmental issues. We identify innovative thinkers and emerging trends in the environmental field. We work with world-renowned experts and authors to develop cross-disciplinary solutions to environmental challenges.

Island Press designs and implements coordinated book publication campaigns in order to communicate our critical messages in print, in person, and online using the latest technologies, programs, and the media. Our goal: to reach targeted audiences—scientists, policymakers, environmental advocates, the media, and concerned citizens—who can and will take action to protect the plants and animals that enrich our world, the ecosystems we need to survive, the water we drink, and the air we breathe.

Island Press gratefully acknowledges the support of its work by the Agua Fund, Inc., Annenberg Foundation, The Christensen Fund, The Nathan Cummings Foundation, The Geraldine R. Dodge Foundation, Doris Duke Charitable Foundation, The Educational Foundation of America, Betsy and Jesse Fink Foundation, The William and Flora Hewlett Foundation, The Kendeda Fund, The Forrest and Frances Lattner Foundation, The Andrew W. Mellon Foundation, The Curtis and Edith Munson Foundation, Oak Foundation, The Overbrook Foundation, the David and Lucile Packard Foundation, The Summit Fund of Washington, Trust for Architectural Easements, Wallace Global Fund, The Winslow Foundation, and other generous donors.

The opinions expressed in this book are those of the author(s) and do not necessarily reflect the views of our donors.